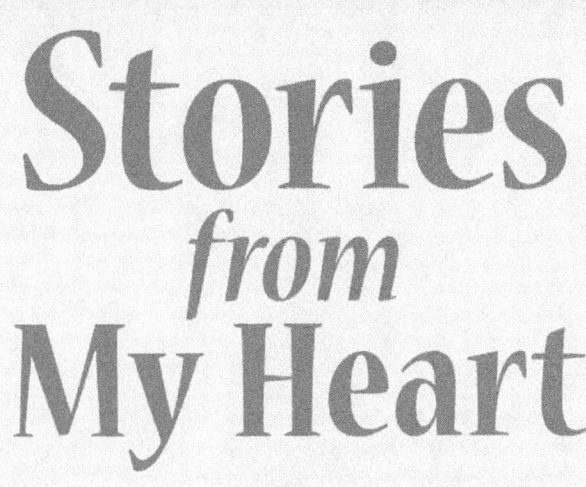

Stories
from
My Heart

♥

*A Cardiologist's
Reflections on the
Gift of Life*

DR. M.P. RAVINDRA NATHAN

STORIES FROM MY HEART

A Cardiologist's Reflections on the Gift of Life

Stories from My Heart is a collection of stories and essays that come right out of the author's heart. These are his real life experiences that depict the fascinating details, challenges, drama and at times humor while working in three different countries on three different continents - India, England and the United States.

Dr. Nathan has been practicing cardiology and internal medicine for the past fifty ears. He has had a remarkable journey in medicine under different conditions in many parts of the world. These collections of well-crafted stories truly portray the triumphs and tragedies in the lives of his patients. The book gives the reader a peek into the twenty first century America as well as a preview of the art of medicine, which is as old as human history itself. All these are compelling stories that touch on various aspects of human lives.

Printed in U. S. A
Some essays first appeared in Medical Economics, Tampa Bay Times, Cortlandt Forum, Journal of Florida Medical Associations and other publications.

ISBN: 1484053583
ISBN-13: 9781484053584

Library of Congress Control Number: 2013906892
CreateSpace Independent Publishing Platform
North Charleston, South Carolina

The physician needs a clear head and a kind heart; the work is arduous and complex, requiring the exercise of the very highest faculties of the mind while constantly appealing to the emotions and finer feelings.

—Sir William Osler, MD

DEDICATION

To my parents, the late Mr. P. Padmanabha Menon and the late Mrs. Ammalu Amma, who constantly encouraged me to excel in everything I do, especially in my studies.

To my loving wife, Susheela Ravindranathan, for her inspiration, guidance, and unflinching support.

To my brother, M. P. Rajappan, BA, BL, IRS, who has been a wonderful mentor and role model throughout my life.

To my sister, Ratnam Sivaraman, who gave me the second gift of life – a kidney transplantation.

ACKNOWLEDGMENTS

I owe a debt of gratitude to the following persons:

Dr. M. V. Pillai, for his advice, encouragement, and the wonderful preface to this book.

Dr. Roy P. Thomas, for his advice and the introduction to the section, "The Art of Medicine."

Dr. Rao Musunuru, my personal cardiologist, for his advice and the introduction to the section, "The Science of Medicine."

Dr. George Thomas, for his invaluable help and the introduction to the section, "The Business and Politics of Medicine."

Helen Gallagher, for her valuable advice, initial review, and endorsement of the book.

My two children, Sandeep and Sandra, both physicians, for their constructive criticism and helpful suggestions. They have always been a great delight in my life.

CONTENTS

About *Stories from My Heart: A Cardiologist's Reflections on the Gift of Life*

The commitment to a career as a doctor is a long journey through medical school, internship, residency, and a full medical practice. *Stories from My Heart: A Cardiologist's Reflections on Life* is an inspiring collection of essays from Dr. Ravindra Nathan's long career in medicine, built around heart-warming stories of his work to help and heal his patients. In reading these essays, collected by Dr. Nathan over fifty years of service to his patients, one realizes what matters most to him when sitting with a patient is his strong passion to save lives.

In *Stories from My Heart* we follow Dr. Nathan's experiences through personal essays that range from working in difficult conditions early in his career in India to serving as a cardiologist on staff at America's top hospitals. Through it all he captures the drama, challenges, and triumphs with great compassion, fascinating details, and humor where it can be found even during tragic situations. As each essay unfolds, the reader moves faster and faster to absorb the details. It is as though we are with Dr. Nathan and his patients during these dramatic life stories.

Few essay collections ring so true and remind us of the fragile nature of life. We are empowered by the efforts of his work, the rewards of good health, and the power of hope and prayers. Dr. Nathan continues to be a source of inspiration to hundreds of people in his clinical practice. By sharing these stories of his life's work he provides the same comfort to us all. There is no better example of a human interest story than those in this thoughtful essay collection.

Helen Gallagher
Author of *Release Your Writing: Book Publishing Your Way* and *Blog Power & Social Media Handbook*,
Book reviewer, national speaker, and member of American Society of Journalists and National Book Critics Circle

Rudyard Kipling's famous first lines in The Ballad of East and West (1889) are often quoted with the incorrect interpretation when one reads only the first few words: "East is East, and West is West, and never the twain shall meet."

Kipling meant a message altogether different if one reads the poem in its entirety. The differences between the East and the West can indeed bring about a lot of positive synergy in human endeavors as exemplified by Steve Jobs who attributed the success of Apple products to an effective blending of India's culture of intuitive thinking to Western technology. Throughout the pages of this magnificent work, Dr. M. P. Ravindra Nathan reinforces that brilliant concept, highlighting how the experiential knowledge and exemplary cognitive skills he learned from India equipped him to transform the gadget-oriented, business-driven, often unfriendly and faceless American medical science into a fine art of healing when professional excellence is blended with empathy, humaneness, and social commitment.

Dr. Nathan is an amazing storyteller who writes with fervor and inimitable fascination for the human spirit. He is endowed with a natural gift for interweaving cutting-edge medical technology with lucid and concise literary finesse. The book is sure to resonate clearly with medicos of yesterday, today, and tomorrow as well as the general public.

M. V. Pillai, MD, FACP
Clinical Professor of Oncology
Kimmel Cancer Centre, Thomas Jefferson University
Philadelphia, PA 19107
Phone : 215 955 3973
Fax: 215 503 3408

The practice of medicine is interesting and exciting, but at times quite challenging and even exasperating. Each day is different in the life of a physician, and there is no clue what is in store for you as you drive to the hospital in the morning.

Some days, the intensive care unit (ICU), coronary care unit (CCU), and emergency department (ED) can be very busy with complex cases that are difficult to manage. There is high-wire drama almost everywhere in the hospital—acute heart attack needing immediate thrombolytic therapy or transfer to the cardiac catheterization laboratory for primary angioplasty, the emergency response team resuscitating someone in cardiac arrest, ventilators hissing away needing constant monitoring, post-surgical cases returning from the operating room (OR) and looking for a bed in the ICU, irate relatives wanting to know how their loved ones are doing, and much more. Then there are rounds to be made on other floors where patients are waiting impatiently to be discharged, the exercise lab looking for you for tests to be completed, the noninvasive lab paging you to read a few stat echoes and EKGs, and at times the emergency room insisting that you see a consultation before leaving to the office.

In addition to all these, on certain days there are special procedures like permanent pacemaker insertion or right heart catheterization or transesophageal echocardiograms (TEE) to be fitted into the schedule too. Because I am not an interventional cardiologist I am spared the demands from the cardiac catheterization lab. And by 11:00 a.m., the office secretary pages, "Where are you? There are three patients already waiting, and you know we have a long day."

Even after office hours there is more work to be done. My box at the heart center will be overflowing with echocardiograms and EKGs to be read and requests for new consults to be seen. Family physicians are waiting to hear from me about their patients who had undergone various cardiac tests during the day, medical records to be completed, and more. Finally, when I get home, there are family matters that need urgent attention.

However, amid all these demands, physicians continue to do their job for one reason: the humanism, the passion that burns inside that encourages them to do what they do—care for patients and save lives. When a patient gets better and goes home with a grateful smile, the satisfaction and pride are the doctor's rewards.

My medical journey started when I was a fourteen-year-old ninth grader. My father opened a small private compounding and dispensing pharmacy in two rooms of our small house after he retired as a compounder (pharmacist) from the government service in Kerala, India. I was his young assistant and substituted for him when he had to urgently step out of the pharmacy. So I got an early introduction to the sights, sounds and smells of diseases and drugs.

My medical school training in Trivandrum, India, and subsequently in various hospitals in England and then in the United States gave me a global experience in health care delivery and the practice of medicine. Working in a suburban community like Brooksville, Florida, certainly has given me enough time to interact with patients and families and get better insight into the complexities of their lives than if I were working in a large city hospital, where physicians are often too busy and have very little time to explore the family dynamics of their own patients. I never looked at any patient as another case on my list; I always saw him or her as an individual with all the human frailties and emotional needs.

The stories in this book have been culled from my experiences in internal medicine and cardiology that stretch over a period of fifty years, spanning three countries on three continents—India, England, and America. These are compelling stories that touch on various aspects of human lives. Some of them are quite personal, one about my own health problem and another about the untimely demise of a young neighbor. I have included one travel story that was quite memorable for the sheer magnitude of problems I encountered during the journey. The names have been changed in a few of the stories to protect the privacy of the persons involved.

The book is divided into three sections to reflect the themes contained in the stories: The Art of Medicine, The Science of Medicine, and The Business and Politics of Medicine. Each section is preceded by a brief introduction from a renowned physician practicing in the US who has special insight and knowledge in that specific area.

Writing and publishing one's experiences and then compiling them into a book amid a busy practice and equally busy family life is not easy. Although in the making for more than two years I am glad the book has finally come out in print. The journey has often been lonely and time consuming but it has all been worthwhile.

"Stories from My Heart" is intended for both the medical and non-medical audience. I sincerely hope you enjoy reading it.

M. P. Ravindra Nathan, MD, FACC
FACP, FRCP (London and Canada), FAHA

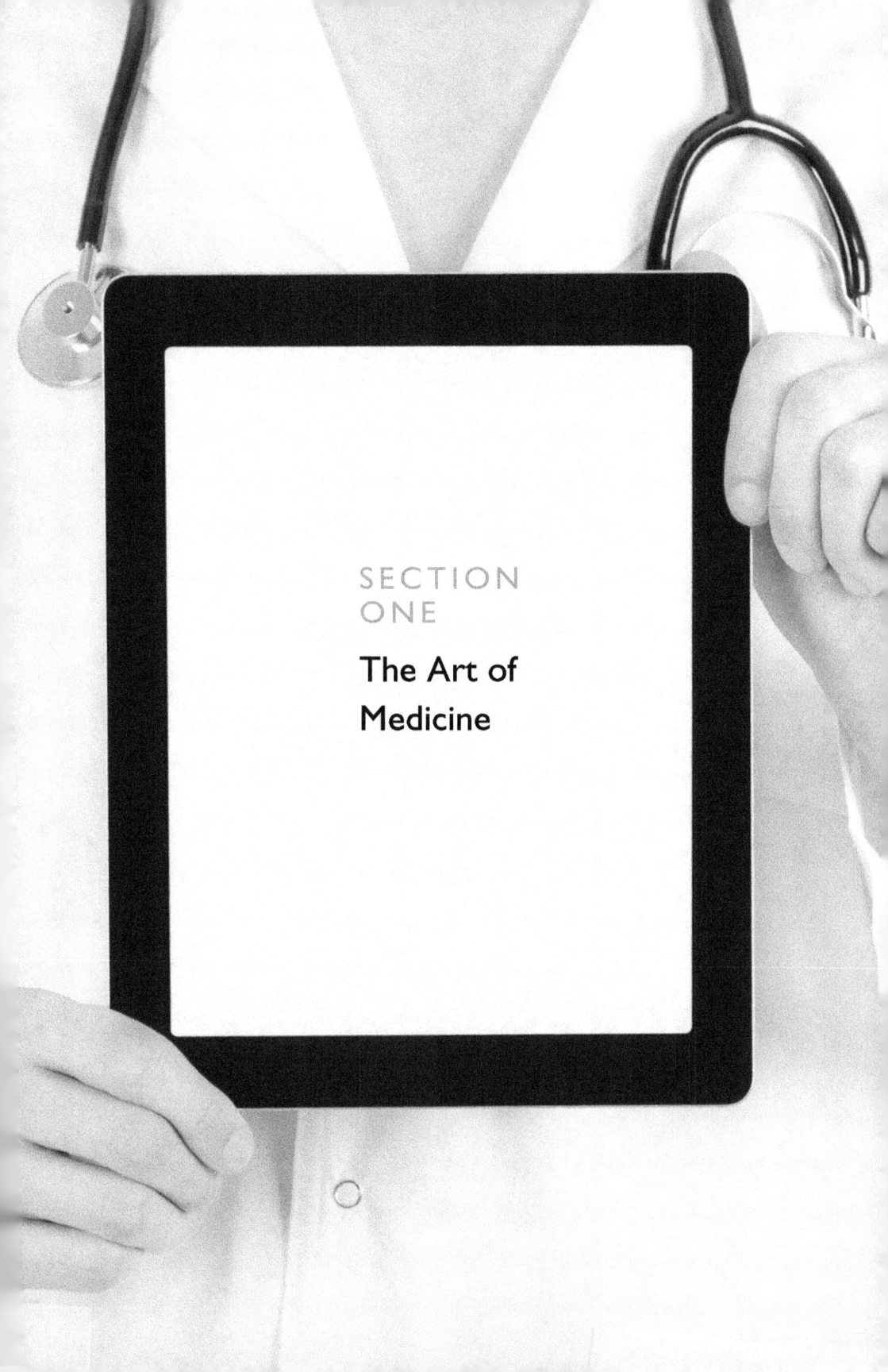

SECTION
ONE

The Art of
Medicine

The Art of Medicine

Stories from My Heart is a collection of essays by Dr. M. P. Ravindra Nathan, an eminent cardiologist practicing in Florida for fifty years. His book gives the reader a peek into the medicine of twenty-first century America as well as a preview of the art of medicine, which is as old as human history itself. Hippocrates said, "Wherever the art of medicine is loved, there is also love of humanity."

In the chapter "My Close Call, Your Wake-Up Call," the author shares his thoughts on life and death. As a busy physician he thought he couldn't afford to get sick, especially on Tuesdays, when his schedule was booked solid. But he had a heart attack on a Tuesday, and Dr. Nathan remembers, "My heart attack made me realize that life happens in the present. Every day now, I live in conscious appreciation of the gift of life."

Dr. Nathan believes in "Prescribing Hope" Unexplained by medical science, some of his patients, presumed terminally ill, continue to lead quality lives for many years.

"An Unscheduled Stop: The Story of a Successful House Call" is a story about an elderly man who came under his care in India after a house call. He was found at home in a deep coma by his relatives. There were definite signs of irreversible brain damage. The family declined hospital admission and wanted him to die peacefully at home. Dr. Nathan gave him general supportive care only and expected him to die soon. But to his surprise, the man walked into his office a few weeks later! Dr. Nathan confesses that to this day he doesn't know how that happened.

About these experiences, he writes, "Medicine is also an art, and many other factors must be considered. Along with the body, the mind also has boundless potential; when used properly it can aid in the healing process."

In "Last Stop" he writes about Margaret, an old woman in a nursing home. "I saw the shattered heart of an old woman stuck in a nursing home, where she was withering away in loneliness. Once she was a lovely daughter, then a passionate wife, later a caring mother, and finally a doting grandmother. Now she has no more roles to play."

Dr. Nathan shows that in such situations the best medicine is inspiring hope in them.

"When a twenty-three-year-old asks to die," what should he do? Angela had been diagnosed with AIDS two years earlier. This was her second episode of pneumocystis pneumonia. She was in severe pain and discomfort with no hope for recovery. She wanted the ventilator that sustained her life turned off. She had the legal right to ask to stop the life support and end her unbearable misery.

"For a moment I tried to put myself in her position," Dr. Nathan writes. "In fact, only a few months ago I had to undergo a major surgery. Just before I went under anesthesia, I had a sudden surge of emotions. What if I didn't wake up after surgery? I could see some of the events in my life especially from childhood, parading in front of my eyes. Perhaps Angela was also reminiscing about childhood memories, her relations with people important in her short life, the many unfinished jobs, and unrealized dreams."

But she wanted to end it all. Apart from giving tender loving care, Dr. Nathan had no further options but to sign the DNR order, which gave her permission to make the final exit with dignity.

Cure sometimes, treat often, comfort always. That is the age-old dictum in medicine. Shakespeare asked the physician in Macbeth, "Canst thou not minister to a mind diseased?" Dr. Nathan says he sometimes feels like a pastor when he ministers to the mind.

As a heart specialist, when he hears a patient complain of chest pain, Dr. Nathan always asks himself, *Are these pains truly from the heart?*

The story of fifty-year-old Maureen with chest pain is typical. On closer look, it turned out that her chest pain was not from her coronaries; her heart was aching for her only son, twenty-eight-year-old Larry, who had returned to her after five years away from home...with full-blown AIDS! Dr. Nathan counseled and helped her to take care of her son during his last days. When Maureen returned to Dr. Nathan after Larry's death, her chest pain was long gone. She was forever grateful to him that she got a chance to be there for Larry, when he needed her most.

But this book is not about blood and tears alone. In "Humor at the Office" we find laughter that is so infectious and contagious. Dr. Nathan liberally gives it to his patients. Unlike infections, it boosts the immune system, diminishes the pain, and reduces the stress.

Hope and hopelessness, pain and joy, illness and recovery are all part of the landscape where a physician dwells.

The art of medicine transcends the science of medicine. Patients facing death or disability turn to a physician for answers, and the physician looks deep into his or her own soul for the right answers. Here the physician is transformed from a repair technician to the healer practicing the timeless, noble craft of medicine. Dr. Nathan's *Stories from My Heart* is an eloquent testimony to that which is still the very best in medicine.

Roy P. Thomas, MD
Roy P Thomas, MD, has practiced internal medicine in Chicago since 1975. He is a prolific writer, an eloquent speaker, and a community leader. He frequently appears on Indian television, giving medical information and advice. He has produced 480 television episodes on different medical topics which are telecast to seventy-two countries. He is well known among the Indian community in North America for his wit, humor, and scholarship

CHAPTER 1

Why Was Arthur Not Getting Better?

The patient seemed blasé about his critical health problems. In truth, he was acting more out of shame than indifference.

When Arthur Clarke first presented in the ED (emergency department), he was in heart failure. At only fifty-eight, this strapping former New York City police officer had an enlarged heart and severe left ventricular dysfunction. An echocardiogram showed a very low ejection fraction of 25 percent.

It turned out that Mr. Clarke (not his real name) was suffering from a chronic cardiac disease called dilated cardiomyopathy. Whether this was an idiopathic condition or a consequence of his moderate alcohol consumption, I couldn't be sure. With good medical care he improved, shed a few pounds, and was soon ready to go home. Medications were adjusted, dietary instructions were given, and he appeared to be on his way to recovery.

A few days later, he was back in the ED complaining of palpitations. This time we diagnosed ventricular tachycardia, a nearly fatal rhythm of the heart if not treated quickly. He needed immediate defibrillation and was stabilized further in the CCU. Before he was discharged I prescribed amiodarone, the effective but costly antiarrhythmic drug, and asked if he could fill and refill the prescription as needed. "No problem, Doc, I'm on my wife's insurance plan, which covers drugs," he said. About weight reduction, he bragged, "I'm going to lose thirty pounds in three months. You just wait."

The next month I saw him in my office for a follow-up visit. He looked well, although at 270 pounds, he was a mere three pounds lighter than he was the last time I'd seen him. And that small weight reduction was probably attributable to the diuretics he was taking.

Just after two weeks Mr. Clarke showed up in the ED, complaining of dizziness and chest discomfort. Again, we had to treat him for recurrent ventricular tachycardia, and this time I referred him to an electrophysiologist for a special study to evaluate the possible origin of this arrhythmia and implantation of an ICD (implantable cardiovertor defibrillator that will quickly deliver a small shock and correct the arrhythmia).

Another two weeks went by, and I spoke with him in my office. "Do I have to take this 'ammodiarone' or whatever you call it, now that I have this gadget?" he asked, pointing to the left side of his chest.

"Yes, you do," I replied. "Otherwise, your ICD will discharge frequently. You know what that is? They are small shocks and not so pleasant. You don't want that."

He was put on a maintenance dose of amiodarone. With ICD and amiodarone, he should be OK now, I thought. But I was wrong. Not long afterward, there was that all too familiar call from the ED.

"Your man is here with the same problem," the ED doctor informed me. "He's had a few more bouts of ventricular tachycardia, and the ICD discharged twice."

"That's strange," I said. "He was well controlled on his medications."

When I saw Arthur in the CCU he appeared shaken. "What happened, Arthur?" I asked. "I didn't expect to see you so soon."

"Oh, Doc, I'm scared. And I've a confession to make."

"What is it? Have you started drinking again?"

"Oh, no. I stopped the amiodarone weeks ago. It's expensive, Doc."

"But you have insurance coverage for prescription drugs, right?"

"I did. But my wife doesn't work anymore, so we have no health insurance now," he admitted.

"Why didn't you tell me?"

"Frankly, I was embarrassed to admit that I didn't have enough money to buy medicine. Can you dig up some from the hospital pharmacy to help me get by?"

So that's what was going on here, I told myself. Arthur was deeply concerned about his health, but he was too proud to ask for help in securing the lifesaving medicine he needed. "Sorry, Arthur, we can't do that. But I can help you get Medicaid benefits."

First, though, we needed to get him at least three weeks' worth of medications, so he could get through until he got his Medicaid card.

I consulted our hospital social worker, and we went to work. First we asked the hospital administrator to come up with some money quickly. He got $100. That was given to a local charitable organization, which would buy amiodarone for Arthur when he showed up with my prescription. I didn't want to hand him the money, fearing that he'd spend it on something other than medicine. He ultimately went home with thirty pills (one month's supply) and a big grin on his face. A month later, his Medicaid card came in the mail.

More than a year has passed, and I haven't seen Arthur in the ED.

Often seemingly noncompliant patients are too proud to admit that they simply can't afford lifesaving medications. If you take the time to inquire into their circumstances, you might be rewarded with surprisingly useful information. You'll then be able to give patients the help they need.[1]

CHAPTER 2

The Final Act of Love

For one patient it was the final act of love to fellow human beings and a unique chance for an extension of her life.

On a Sunday morning in May two years ago I got a stat page.

There were only three patients in the hospital to make rounds, so I was looking forward to a game of tennis in the afternoon. Although it was only early spring, many of my patients had already left Brooksville for their summer residences in the north. Here, in Florida, we call them the "snow birds." They flock to the emergency rooms in winter, so we are always very busy at that time. They begin to leave the area for their northern residences by April; therefore, summer brings a little respite, which we always welcome. The ED, however, had begun to feel the pinch, and the hospital census had started to plummet. The director of nursing was worried; she would have to lay off a few nurses if this "drought" continued.

Then I got a stat call from the medical ICU. Dr. Jerry Sanders, one of my cardiology colleagues, wanted me to insert a Swan-Ganz catheter into the lungs in a patient of his, Marion, admitted the day before with a heart attack.

"Why can't you do it yourself?" I asked.

"Oh, this is for the transplant team. People from Life Link are here."

Ours is a small community hospital, and we don't do any transplant surgery. So I knew some dying patient must have filled out the organ donation card. Life Link in Tampa coordinates all transplant surgeries in our area, and the team members arrive on the scene when organs are ready to be harvested

"They want a line to be inserted to monitor and stabilize her condition before she is taken to the OR. They just told me the treating cardiologist can't do it—some crazy insurance rules, I suppose," he added.

Now the story unfolded. Marion, only fifty-two years old, was admitted with chest pains the day before, which turned out to be an acute myocardial infarction. She came to the ER in good time, during the "window of opportunity" and was eligible for the wonder drug, tPA, a clot-buster. "This drug will open up the blocked coronary artery, so it would be lifesaving," she was told.

Tissue plasminogen activator (tPA) is a drug that dissolves the unwanted clots that are commonly associated with heart attacks and strokes. When infused within the first four hours of a heart attack the results are good. By quickly breaking down the clots, a process called *thrombolysis,* it restores the flow in the coronary artery, contains the heart attack, and reduces the ultimate damage.

Unfortunately, the outcome was quite different. Poor Marion developed a headache during the night shortly after she received the tPA, and she became lethargic by morning. "Oh, my God, I hope she is not having a stroke," one of the nurses exclaimed in a terrified voice. We had had our share of strokes following thrombolytic treatment in this small community. No matter how much explanation you give, the family becomes inconsolable when such a devastating complication occurs. Pretty soon everybody sprang into action. An emergency CT scan of the brain showed massive bilateral cerebral hemorrhage. Marion's breathing became labored, and she had to be put on a ventilator. The neurologist tiptoed in later and looked at the EEG. "Brain dead" was his solemn comment.

The family was shocked on hearing the news, naturally, unable to fathom this rapid turn of events. A vibrant middle-aged woman just a few hours ago, Marion was now clinging to her dear life; it would be just a matter of time. John, her husband, kept a constant vigil throughout the night, watching a struggling coterie of nurses, doctors, and technicians fumbling around Marion without much success. He wanted to see me, although I was not the treating cardiologist.

It was one of the most difficult moments in my life. We looked at each other with mixed emotions; neither of us could utter a single word. He appeared to be initially stunned, then agitated, later confused, and finally tears started trickling down from his eyes. The sequence of events was too fast for his comprehension. I took his hand gently and led him to the small prayer room adjacent to the medical ICU and sat down with him.

Slowly he opened up and started telling me how loving and helpful Marion had been throughout her life, and how he and the children adored her. More than a wife, she was also his business partner, bookkeeper, and confidante. She didn't deserve a fate like this. He kept looking at me with melancholic eyes. He didn't know how he was going to cope.

I wanted to recite something from *Bhagawad Geeta*, the Hindu scripture, wherein the Lord says, "It is all one's Karma, or destiny. Don't grieve for the living or the departed. Leave everything to Me." Conceptually simple, those are hard words to say to a man who sees a lonely life with its attendant travails and rigors looming in front of him.

Ever since we started using thrombolytics for acute heart attacks, every cardiologist in my community has seen one of his cases going sour with this dreadful complication. Thankfully, the numbers have been low. A couple of years ago I had my terrifying experience too, when Jerome, a sixty-four-year-old who received the clot-buster, developed a stroke and eventually died. While talking to his wife in the emergency room, I had assigned a possibility of one percent for this potential twist, and the wife readily gave her consent to administer the drug. She expected her husband to come home in a week, all cured.

Although a lot of decisions in clinical practice are made on a scientific basis, the results can still be inexplicably variable. In spite of extensive research, clinical trials, and our own experience and expertise, complications do occur. I guess we cannot escape our own fallibilities, and our learning is never complete.

In Marion's case, the only job left was to finish the paperwork and contact the Life Link team who was always ready. The husband gave his consent for donation of her organs. The energetic nurses from the transplant team, Hahn and Sheryl, arrived promptly and appeared to be very eager to get on with preliminary work. And I went ahead with the last cardiac intervention in her life.

I knew the procedure had to be done very carefully and with absolute sterility. The organs soon would be going to different people in Florida, all eagerly awaiting their gifts of life. Hahn was ready to start his inguinal lymph node biopsy. The technician was already drawing the blood, filling up several red-, green-, and purple-topped tubes for tissue typing and cross matching. Usually I am excited to do this procedure, but this time it was simply to prime her up before she was taken to the operating room for the ultimate 'harvest.' Her fluid balance was maintained and cardiac, respiratory, and renal statuses were stabilized. And Marion, barely living, went for the ultimate surgery about midnight, without any fanfare. Her liver, kidneys, pancreas, and small bowel went to different people eagerly waiting a beeper's call away for their turn on the computer.

"You know John, your wife is going to help a lot of people today. Life is eternal," I said, quoting again from *Bhagavad Gita*, trying to hide the tears in my eyes. He looked relieved and at peace as I left the room.

For poor Marion, it was the final act of love to fellow human beings and a unique chance for an extension of her life. And thanks to her, a few people could celebrate an early Christmas.[2]

[2] First published in *Practice Perspective*, the Journal of the Florida Medical Association. July 2003, pg 17.

CHAPTER 3

Those Pills Are Too Costly, Doctor!

The author strongly believes we owe it to ourselves to find ways to help pa-tients procure prescription drugs to ensure their compliance.

One of the most common questions I encounter when I hand over the prescription to a patient at the end of the office visit is "How much is this going to cost me?"

Recently, Bill, a sixty-six-year-old patient of mine with heart disease, diabetes, and high cholesterol levels, sent me a neatly typed note that said:

"Dear Dr. Nathan, The co-pay on my drugs is getting very expensive for me. You know I am on several of them. I would like to take generic drugs instead of those costly brand names. Here is the list and the price for a ninety-day supply." The drugs included: 1. Actos Tabs 30 mg $35, 2. Zocor Tabs 40 mg $35, 3. Avapro Tabs 150 mg $35, 4. Catapres TTS 0.2 mg $35, 5. Novolin 70/30 Insulin $35.

"Can you tell me if I can get cheaper alternatives that will save me some money?"

While I was trying to understand his problem, in came Janet, a very sensible and compliant woman, for her routine follow-up. She said to me, "Dr. Nathan, I get just six hundred sixty-five dollars a week, that's all. How can I afford this expensive drug for cholesterol? It costs nearly three dollars a pill! Is there a cheaper version?"

My biggest headache came from Henry, seventy-five years old, who showed up in the emergency room with increasing shortness of breath for the umpteenth time. It had taken me several months to stabilize his heart failure from severe dilated cardiomyopathy. Finally with a combination of five drugs, he could stay out of the hospital for the longest period in his recent life, i.e., four months.

Now he was back in the ER. Putting his fragile pride aside, he confessed that he didn't have the money to buy Coreg, a costly but effective drug. He only had Medicaid for his insurance. Then I had to call the drug company and put him on an indigent drug program, so he could get coupons for free drugs. And once again, he got better.

Do these stories sound familiar? Actually, the imbalance between the cost of drugs and affordability has become glaringly obvious these days. Most of my patients are retirees living on a limited income, and a good 30 percent of them do not have any prescription plan. With the prices of drugs soaring every day, they need some help. Everybody is concerned that patients will shortchange their medical care for a price break. I have learned one thing after nearly five decades of medical practice. Compliance, to a large extent, is directly related to affordability.

One day, the local Pfizer pharmaceutical representative came on his usual monthly visit to my office. Since we use a lot of their drugs, especially Lipitor and Norvasc, I asked him what he could do for my less-wealthy patients. "Oh, I am glad you asked the question," he said. "But first, I must ask you something. Do you know how much it costs us to put a drug in the market? Take a guess."

I shook my head. I didn't know the answer.

"Eight hundred million dollars!" he said. A long pause. "So you know why these drugs are so costly. But we have now launched a discount program to all the eligible senior citizens."

"Really? This is great news. Our practice primarily consists of Medicare folks," I said.

"Get your patients to fill out a form if they are below an annual gross income of eighteen thousand dollars for individuals and twenty-four thousand dollars for couples. Actually, you can send your patients to any of the participating pharmacies and they will get them a special card called the Pfizer Share Card. Then, they need to pay only fifteen dollars for three months' supply. There may be a little paperwork involved, that is all," he said reassuringly.

When I called Janet the next day and asked about her income, she said: "Are you kidding? My income is way below that amount!" So I asked her to go to the pharmacy and fill out applications for as many companies as possible that provide these share cards. Other companies are also warming up to this innovative trend. GlaxoSmithKline has launched their special "Free Orange Card" and Novartis has joined suit. Eli Lilly also has recently announced their plans to subsidize medicines to low-income seniors. With these cards one can save about 30 percent off the regular price. Actually Merck has gone one step further. With a doctor's prescription and a special application form given by the doctor, one can even get the drugs free for one year. How can you beat that?

In addition, many company reps bring discount coupons to the office on their routine visits, and my nurse hands them over to the patients as needed. We have displayed them at the nurse's station in a prominent fashion. I am also keeping track of the drugs that are going off patent; recently Vasotec, Prilosec, Prozac, and Claritin have gone off patent. In addition, a lot of our poor patients get free samples from our well-stocked medicine cupboard, which they call jokingly "People's Pharmacy."

Since the Bush administration's 2001 proposal for a Medicare discount card may not become a reality any time soon, this new initiative to improve access to prescription drugs for the financially strapped Medicare population by prominent drug companies is admirable. In small steps, these companies are trying to address the problem of skyrocketing drug costs. It is not clear if these programs will solve the problem but it is a welcome start.

European governments seem to be able to set price controls on drugs, and some drugs are 40 percent cheaper than in the US. And most governments typically reimburse prescription drug costs under state-sponsored health care systems. In the US, marketing costs maybe one major factor driving up the costs.

I strongly believe we owe it to ourselves to find ways to help patients procure prescription drugs to ensure their compliance. Many years ago Sir William Osler said, "It is much more important to know what sort of a patient has a disease than what sort of a disease a patient has." Thinking along the same lines, the modern physician should ask what kind of finances the patient has before prescribing (costly) drugs. Now it is up to the Congress to institute a comprehensive drug coverage program for all, especially for our senior citizens.[3]

[3] First published in *Practice Perspectives*, Quarterly journal of the Florida Medical Association, January 2003, pg 29.

CHAPTER 4

A Case of Threatened Abortion!

The use of a new drug gave a lot of anxiety to the doctor, but all is well that ends well.

The year was 1972. Shortly after finishing my postgraduate training in medicine in England, I returned to my home state of Kerala, India, and took up a position as assistant attending physician in a large county hospital. Fresh from training in some of the good hospitals in London, Cambridge, Sunderland and Sheffield and with an academic bent, I was eager to do a little clinical research, especially since clinical materials were plentiful here.

One day, Annie, aged twenty-five years, presented with abdominal pain at three months of gestation. There was also some questionable vaginal spotting. This was a precious baby, since she had a history of two prior abortions. Dr. Mary Antony, her obstetrician, was very concerned. Not wanting to take any chances, she admitted Annie to the maternity ward with a tentative diagnosis of threatened abortion and put her on complete bed rest, fluid diet, and close observation.

I had just started doing a phase III clinical trial on a brand-new anthelmintic drug called Tetramisole. It was touted to be potentially the best drug for ascariasis (roundworm infestation in the belly). And indeed, ascariasis was a common third world parasitosis in those days. A lot of our patients were poor and indeed suffered from this infestation. Half of the children who queued up in pediatric clinic each day were successfully de-wormed. Just like the annual children's physicals in America, most children in India, especially from poor families, got routine anthelmintic treatment every year. And they would brag during their next clinic visit about how many worms they passed!

The protocol for my roundworm research was simple. I would go around the various floors and collect stool samples from patients with abdominal discomfort. My lab technician examined the stool and did a roundworm ova count by the McMaster method, a standard technique for estimating the number of ova per gram in a given sample. If the count was high, suggesting heavy infestation, that patient would be included in the trial. Initially, only pediatric patients were enrolled, but later adults were also included. The nurses began praising this drug as they became aware of its efficacy. And many older patients came forward to be tested and treated voluntarily.

Annie's stool sample reached the lab, and the technician informed me that she satisfied the eligibility criteria for the trial. However, I was skeptical about treating Annie with the new drug.

"Doesn't this woman have a threatened abortion? How will the drug affect her pregnancy?" I asked Dr. Antony.

"I don't know, Doctor. This is a new drug after all," she said. "You know better about it than I do. It is your call." She tossed the responsibility back to me.

Anyway, I decided this one little pill was not going to hasten her abortion, and there appeared to be enough roundworm ova in her stool to justify giving the pill. There was no mention of this complication in the literature, although the total number of publications on the drug was just a handful at that time. Annie got the standard dose, just one small pill.

That night, I slept fitfully, thinking about what terrible things could happen to her pregnancy from the pill. And if something did go wrong,

I would hear plenty of corridor talk like, "Look what that hotshot from England did to poor Annie's baby!"

The following morning, as I walked onto her floor with my heart in my hand, the nurse came running to me excitedly and announced in Malayalam, our native language, *"Doctarey, you know what? Annie is passing a bunch of worms!"* Awkward animations and facial contortions added some spunk to her narration. I glanced toward Annie's bedside. It was screened off with a portable three-sided partition, commonly used for privacy in those days in a general ward holding some thirty patients. There were not many private bathrooms available for each ward in this poor government hospital. Annie was glued to the bedside commode.

Before the nurse disposed of the contents of the commode, I took a peek. Sure enough, it was full of slimy, wriggly balls of roundworms. The drug surely did its job! Now we waited for any possible complications while I prayed hard and held my breath. Annie looked at me with a puzzled and admiring expression, "Did all those come from my belly?"

I returned her glance and nodded my head. Yes, Annie, they did. But I hope your baby is safe and sound."

Within twenty-four hours, Annie announced with a wide grin that her bellyache was completely gone, and she was ready to go home! Dr. Antony was immensely pleased that there were no signs of miscarriage. But only after Annie's safe delivery of a healthy baby a few months later, could I really rest easy.

Tetramisole became an instant "celebrity" in our hospital, as Annie's story spread by word-of-mouth in that small community. And I earned the dubious reputation as the "roundworm doctor."[4]

[4] First published in the Journal of the Florida Medical Association, January 2006, page 12.

CHAPTER 5

My Hurricane Experiences

Hurricanes are purveyors of perils, so beware! And living in Florida, the author had to face the daunting challenges from nature's wrath.

May 1, 2006

While I was watching the CNN news, the weatherman suddenly materialized on the screen to give this forecast: twenty-seven storms and fifteen hurricanes, seven of them severe, for this year!

"Oh, my!" I said to myself. "Get ready for another year of suffering! Only one more month for the hurricane season to start."

Memories of last year's weather-related fiascos flooded my mind in a flash.

On moving to Florida twenty-five years ago, I was so excited about living and working in the sunshine state and to finally retire without relocating again. I still am, but the events of the last two years have curbed my enthusiasm, just a little. Can you imagine we had a total of twenty-three storms in a span of fifteen months that affected one or another part of Florida? Eight of these turned out to be major and three of them, Katrina, Rita, and Wilma, produced catastrophic damages?

My house in Hernando County, West Central Florida, is at least twenty miles from the Gulf. Although we escaped a direct hit from any storm last year, the preparations for the relentless hurricanes had worn us out. Just when we thought the hurricane season was over, came Wilma. The banks and schools were closed, and a few of my more cautious patients decided to evacuate ahead of time, although our town of Brooksville was only at the periphery of Wilma's potential landfall. But many of our friends and relatives who lived in South Florida were not so lucky.

On Sunday, October 23, 2005, we were tracking the progress of the "big W" on the Weather Channel. Thanks to the accurate eyewitness reporting by the experts, we knew that it was likely to make its landfall in Naples on the west coast of Florida, lose some of its steam, become just Category1 with less potential for major damage, and then course toward Palm Beach County in the east and exit to the Atlantic Ocean. But whoever thought this monster would land as a Category 3 storm?

My sister-in-law, Dr. Sushama (Mini) Venugopal, a pediatrician, and her husband, Dr. C. (Venu) Venugopal, a cardiologist, both practicing in West Palm Beach, decided not to evacuate since the weatherman said it was going to be a "Cat 1 or at the most, 2." "It was not easy to pack up and flee at short notice with the two elderly mothers staying with us," Mini said. My wife and I urged them to evacuate early in order to avoid any potential problems, but they decided to brave it out. After all, they had been through two storms the previous year, Jean and Frances. Storm shutters pulled down, water collected and stored, refrigerators stocked up, cars gassed up and generator ready to run, they felt they were more than prepared. I kept in touch with them constantly, while keeping an eye on the Weather Channel in case the storm decided to make a slight turn to the Tampa Bay area like Charlie did in 2004.

Then came the shocker on Monday morning, October 24, 2005. Wilma, after stalling in Cancun and the Yucatan peninsula for two days, just roared into Southwest Florida at 130 mph, and all hell broke loose. A category three storm! In a six-hour coast-to-coast flight, it killed six people, created widespread damage and destruction to almost everything in its path, besides cutting off electricity for over six million people.

Mini and family were devastated, as were most people in South Florida. About a half hour before it was expected to pass through West Palm Beach, she said over the phone: "I can hear the howling wind, almost like a freight train coming. Looks like it might hit our house any minute!"

Venu added wistfully, "It was foolish not to have evacuated. Too late *now.*"

There was unmistakable panic in his voice. While we were talking, they lost Power and the phone line went dead. Not even cell phones were working with all the towers down. No word for two days. We heard from the news that several trees were uprooted, many buildings suffered major damage, and low-lying areas flooded in Palm Beach County as Hurricane Wilma marched in, but fortunately they escaped the devastation of a storm surge, being quite far away from the Gulf of Mexico.

When he finally called from the hospital, Venu's story was frightening. "All of a sudden the outside noise picked up. I could hear things breaking and banging outside the window. It felt as though a jet plane was about to land on the roof. With the torrential rains, I thought the whole roof would cave in."

Our waterfront condo in Belle Isle, near South Beach, Miami, fortunately had a hurricane shutter for the sliding door facing the ocean, but none for the glass windows in the two bedrooms. Experiencing the storm's fury left our tenant, a young ophthalmology resident, quite shaken. She said: "Wilma blitzed through Belle Isle. I could see this floor-to-ceiling glass window in the bedroom literally bending, ready to give in. My husband and I hid in a closet. The condo below us on the twenty-second floor was ripped apart; the unprotected sliding glass door shattered, the front door flew open, and everything inside was blown into the corridor.

"Luckily, the owners of that condo were in Europe. Several boats anchored at the marina sank; the rest were battered against the wall, a complete loss," she added.

Three days after the storm, I tried to contact my family members again in West Palm Beach. Phone lines were still disrupted. I paged Venu at the hospital. The operator said the hospital was still running on generators. When I asked her if I could drive over and see my folks, she said, "You better check with the police. There is a curfew between 7:00 p.m. and 7:00 a.m. Being a doctor, you may be able to come in, but I wouldn't take the risk. Besides, it is impossible to get gas without waiting for hours in those long lines."

When Venu finally called me back on the fourth day, his words weren't very comforting. "Life is miserable here. No power. There is plenty of gas, but only half a dozen gas stations in this county have generators. The city looks dead. I have never evacuated for a storm before, but this time I really should have. It is not worth the agony and anxiety."

Many of my friends in South Florida bitterly complained that the weatherman underestimated the strength of this storm, and hence they were ill prepared.

"It is still bad out here *Chetta*," said Venu the following day. "No cable TV. Internet services are dead, no cell phone services. Power outages are everywhere. We still don't have power in this area."

So, this is how it will be if a strong hurricane like Wilma hits your area, I reminded myself.

Hurricanes are purveyors of perils. Now I realize living in Florida means one will have to face the daunting challenges from nature's wrath. Every year, when the hurricane season starts, I educate my patients that no matter what's the category, it's always better to take precautions. I tell them to keep a hurricane kit handy and to make a medical checklist that should contain basic details of their illnesses, a list of their medicines with enough supply for a week, recent lab tests if any, and other items. Survival under these arduous conditions, especially for our elderly patients with multiple illnesses, depends on how much preparation they have done beforehand.

As one of my patients who moved from the Sacramento valley in California after an earthquake said, "Doc, here you get at least three days to evacuate, not thirty seconds, so you shouldn't really complain."

"Exactly my feelings too. Yes, this is one good reason to stay put in Florida. I am planning to do just that," I told him.

I sincerely prayed that no hurricanes would come my way any time soon.[5]

---

[5] October 30, 2005

CHAPTER 6

Seeking the Diagnosis, *I Stumbled on the Cure*

A patient encounter that happened thirty years ago is still teaching the author about medicine.

It was a typically grueling session at the outpatient clinic in my home state of Kerala, India. This was my first job after finishing my postgraduate work in 1969, and I was eager to give the locals who visited this large government hospital the benefit of my British training.

By 8:00 a.m. a crowd of patients was already waiting. On days like this, my resident and I would generally see almost three hundred patients in five hours. We'd ask about the chief complaint and do a cursory exam while the patient remained standing. At best, we could only prescribe some stock medicine or an antibiotic from the hospital dispensary. Mercifully, many of the patients' problems were mild, so they didn't require hospitalization. But enough neglected and chronically ill patients came to boost the two-hundred-bed hospital's census to more than three hundred.

When Mr. Jamal arrived surrounded by his wife, three wailing children, and several friends from his village, I could tell that he was one of the seriously ill. His face contorted with pain, he said he'd been experiencing abdominal discomfort, weight loss, and fever for a month. But he had no cough, diarrhea, or bloody stools. And, because of his Islamic faith, I was sure his problems weren't related to alcohol.

Why hadn't he sought help earlier? "Sahib," he told me, "if I don't work one day, my Beebi and three kids will go to bed hungry." He spoke haltingly, clearly divulging something he'd rather have kept to himself.

Mr. Jamal's comment didn't surprise me. His dirty garments and ragtag turban declared his abject poverty. Daily wage laborers like him earned low incomes and simply worked until they dropped dead. Many regarded hospitalization as just one step before the grave, and therefore something they should avoid. Often, friends or neighbors who entered the hospital were carried out in coffins.

Mrs. Jamal's eyes, welling with tears, seemed to plead with me: "*Don't let him die. Do something.*" I fervently hoped that I could, for the family's sake.

Mr. Jamal looked tired and chronically ill. Dehydration had accentuated the lines on his face, making him appear older than his forty-five years. He was frightened, too; his dark, deeply set eyes watched me carefully, and he barely responded to my questions.

I could feel a few small lymph nodes in Mr. Jamal's neck and both axillae, but they didn't seem particularly menacing. He had bad teeth, the result of chewing tobacco; this was a common problem in an area, where there were no dentists to undo the damage.

There was significant hepatomegaly, but no splenomegaly or ascites. A chest X-ray revealed a little hilar prominence, but no TB or cancer. CBC showed mild anemia with no abnormal cells. The few hookworm ova in his stool sample were common for India's barefoot laborers. There were no amebic parasites. The limited liver function tests we could do in those days were unrevealing, and CT and ultrasound technology didn't exist yet.

I pondered the differential diagnosis. Mr. Jamal clearly didn't have pulmonary tuberculosis, the scourge that had taken the lives of thousands of undernourished Indians. Nor did he have a malignancy of the lung or any form of leukemia. Nonalcoholic cirrhosis was a possibility, especially with his poor nutritional status and enlarged liver. Hodgkin's disease and other lymphomas were strong considerations too since they were quite common. But the most likely possibility, I thought, was carcinoma of the liver. Suddenly, my heart ached. The diagnosis of a cancer or lymphoma would be an immediate death sentence for Mr. Jamal. Our government clinic had no facilities for chemotherapy or radiation, and my patient couldn't afford a private cancer center. If he were to die, his entire family would surely starve.

Mr. Jamal needed an urgent workup. A lymph node biopsy might give me an answer, but the busy surgeon wouldn't get to it for a day or two. I knew that with cancer or lymphoma, the pathology was in that enlarged liver. However, liver biopsies were rarely performed in India's community hospitals in those days, because of the possible complications and the lack of adequate blood supply for transfusions. Despite these drawbacks, I decided to do a liver biopsy with a Menghini needle the following day.

With cringing submissiveness, Mr. Jamal stoically tolerated the needle's assault. I prayed that the Lord would keep my inexperienced, trembling hands steady. I worried not about my reputation, but about my conscience. Above all, I wanted to help Mr. Jamal cheat his apparent rendezvous with death.

As I pulled back the syringe's plunger, there was a spurt of chocolate-brown liquid. "Anchovy sauce!" I heard myself exclaim, recalling the metaphor from medical school. My needle had penetrated an abscess cavity, yielding the pus typical of an amebic liver abscess. After the abscess drained, I administered a course of emetine and chloroquine, the best drugs then available.

Mr. Jamal made a complete recovery.

Just as my professors had stressed in medical school, I've learned that most often, we encounter the common diseases in clinical practice— even when the presentation is unusual. Amebiasis is endemic in south India, and, left untreated, it can lead to amebic hepatitis and liver abscess, well-recognized complications. I'd been thrown off track by Mr. Jamal's lack of typical colonic symptoms and by the paucity of ameba in his stool sample. But serendipitously, perhaps because of my headstrong desire to help, I'd given Mr. Jamal the right treatment.

When Mrs. Jamal came to pick up her husband, her three scrawny, shy, but curious kids clinging to her sari, I saw tears of gratitude in her eyes. They seemed to be telling me: *You* did do *something for my husband!* Pondering my incredible luck, I became misty-eyed too. When I'd first met her, I had groped for words to comfort her and wondered how I could justify her faith in me. Now I was relieved that I'd been able to help, and that Mr. Jamal would still be around to support his family.

I knew then that my training in medicine would never end. Nor would the responsibility to alleviate suffering among the most neglected people. To this day, I still treat them at no charge in my practice, and often fondly remember Mr. Jamal.[6]

[6] Reprinted with permission from *Medical Economics*: October 11, 1999, 76:19 pg 152-157. *Medical Economics* is a copyrighted publication of Advanstar Communications, Inc. All rights reserved.

CHAPTER 7

"Doctor, My Chest Is Hurting Badly!"

A chest pain in a patient with established heart disease turns out to be of an entirely different etiology

The ER (emergency room) called me at 3:00 a.m. with a possible admission. I had gone to bed just three hours before, after a long day's work that included a couple of tiresome meetings as well. The ER doctor reminded me, "This is not one of your patients, but you are on call for cardiology." So I had no choice and had to accept the patient to my service.

Clark Mason, a fifty year old gentleman, had presented to the ER earlier with severe chest pain. He said he had undergone a triple vessel coronary artery bypass graft surgery (CABG) in Seattle, Washington. The pain started as he was coming through Brooksville in his small truck. He was going from Georgia to South Florida, and he made this trip frequently, making deliveries to companies. Apparently he had had severe pain for more than an hour, and he decided to pull into the nearest ER, which happened to be our hospital—Brooksville Regional.

The ER physician felt that the patient might be having an acute myocardial infarction (MI), a heart attack. The EKG he faxed to my house showed only mild sinus tachycardia and a minor abnormality called left bundle branch block. These are nonspecific abnormalities but they could mask any possible underlying MI. So I decided that a trip to the ER was

33

unfortunately necessary for further evaluation. Maybe we could even do a primary angioplasty (PTCA) and open up the clogged artery right away, which would save him from the ravages of a heart attack including death!

In the ER, the scene was typical of a patient having an MI, Clark writhing in chest pain and asking for pain medications, the nurse trying to find a vein to start the second IV. The morphine given through the first heparin lock (hep lock) hadn't touched the patient. The ER doctor was standing next to him stroking his forehead and uttering a few comforting words. I found the first hep lock was not working. The nurse wondered if I could put in a CVP line.

When I was looking for sites, I suddenly found that he already had a Groshong, a semipermanent catheter, inserted on the left subclavian region, presumably for frequent IV drug administration. That was surprising since he wasn't undergoing cancer chemotherapy that needed a good IV line for drugs, nor was he suffering from any major gastrointestinal disease that would prevent him from eating or interfere with his digestion. The latter situation usually called for hyperalimentation, or chronic feeding by intravenous method, and would need a Groshong or similar catheter insertion. He appeared to be well built and maybe even a little plump, far from looking like somebody who could be suffering from any conditions that needed a Groshong.

"What is this for?" I asked, pointing to his Groshong.

"Oh, you know I have very difficult veins. After the bypass surgery, they put one in so that I can have medicines in an emergency." He apologized for giving so much trouble at this hour to all of us and constantly thanked me and the nurses.

"That is funny, insert a Groshong for venous access in an otherwise healthy man." I mumbled to myself. "Are you sure that you don't have any other problems—cancer, malabsorption, and such?"

"No, I don't have any other problems. I've had a lot of war injuries, and there is a lot of scar tissue in me," he told me in between his sobs with a crackly voice.

And yet, when I examined him, he wasn't diaphoretic, pale or apprehensive, and not short of breath…just demanding that he get some pain killers. I found that the Groshong wasn't working either, so I tried to get a line through his right subclavian without success. But finally with some difficulty I got one into the right femoral vein and started the whole works with IV nitroglycerine, morphine, IV Lopressor, and more.

After the first morphine, he appeared to show some relief and thanked me profusely. Then I asked him a few more questions.

"So, where did you have the surgery?"

"In that big hospital down by the water in Seattle."

"You don't remember the name of the hospital, Clark?"

"How can I remember all these details? It was five years ago!"

"Do you remember the name of the surgeon?"

"Right now I am very tired and in pain." He didn't even think that my question was pertinent.

"That is funny; you had a major heart surgery, and you don't know the name of the hospital or the surgeon." To this he responded by starting to roll around in pain and grimacing. He asked for more morphine. And he received a second dose in less than ten minutes.

"Tell me, who do you live with? I want to let them know that you are here." He said he lived with his elderly mother in Clearwater and didn't want to let her know. Why? Because the news of him being in the hospital would kill her! More stories emerged shortly. He was divorced and had two children who were living with his ex-wife. He was visiting his girlfriend in Georgia with whom he had three children two, five, and eight years old. He didn't want us to call them either. But to the nurse, he said that he had seven children all together. He wouldn't give the telephone number of anybody and wouldn't show even the driver's license in his wallet! I couldn't quite understand such secrecy!

In the ICU, it was more of the same; he was constantly rolling around in pain. The first set of cardiac enzymes was normal. No new EKG changes. But he was constantly demanding morphine. He complained to one nurse that nobody was doing anything for him. His tone had become different now; no more apologies, no more nice talk. He even suggested to the nurse when I was out of the ICU that we put him on a PCA pump (for continuous infusion of morphine, which he could adjust himself)!

"A PCA pump," I exclaimed in total bewilderment. "How do you even know about a PCA pump? You couldn't remember the name of your hospital or surgeon." To which he didn't answer but pointed to his chest and said, "I am having spasms right here. They come in waves. Do something about it, will you?"

"I need to talk to your mother. Can you give me her phone number?"

"I don't want you to bother her."

"Why this secrecy, may I ask?"

He appeared to be visibly upset. Later the nurse called me aside and said that he was demanding some injection or other all the time and kept on asking for more morphine. His stories were inconsistent. Someone from the social services department came later, tried to break his code of secrecy, but couldn't get anything more out of him. There were all kinds of stories floating around. One nurse even hinted that he might have a shady past.

"How do we know if he is not a mass murderer? He even has that look!" one nurse suggested.

"Oh, I didn't know that they came with special looks!" I tried to lighten the situation.

Since he had so much pain, an abnormal EKG, and a history to go with possible unstable angina, I felt we should take him to cardiac cath lab and study him. I explained the minimal risks involved in the procedure. He readily agreed, almost welcoming the suggestion, and he remarked, "I am worried if any of those pipes in my heart are blocked again." Then he asked for more morphine because, "those wicked pains have started again."

At this time I went to his room and asked if he could remember the name of his previous hospital, to which he again answered in the negative. I was beginning to think that we might have a real morphine addict on our hands.

"We need to study the surgical details and hookup of the by-pass grafts before we can do another cardiac cath." I tried to explain.

Clearly he didn't like our postponing the heart cath and became visibly upset.

"Give me my clothes," he demanded.

"Where are you going?" Actually, I wanted to ask him if he was going hospital shopping but didn't.

"You don't believe me, do you? You think that I am some kind of a phony, right?"

I wanted to say "right" but decided to simply advise him why he shouldn't discharge against medical advice at that time. He had already worked himself into an angry mood, got up, dressed himself, and walked out of the ICU.

Mr. Mason clearly knew that we were on to his case. There was not even an inkling of pain on his face!

"Long live, cardiac Munchausen!" I exclaimed to myself.

Munchausen syndrome is a type of mental illness, a psychiatric factitious disorder, in which the patient acts like he or she is constantly symptomatic from whatever disease he or she is feigning and continues to demand medications for relief. Those who present with abdominal pain of an emotional type even voluntarily subject themselves for unnecessary surgery, sometimes multiple surgeries. They don't mind undergoing painful treatment, risky tests, or surgery.

Named for Baron von Munchausen, an eighteenth-century German officer who was known for embellishing the stories of his life and experience, this syndrome is perhaps the most severe type of factitious illness. These patients go from hospital to hospital in the same area or in the state; sometimes they even go searching for hospitals nationally. Some of them have been known to hunt for hospitals in other countries and occasionally other continents as well!

I remember reading about a few instances in which the same patient got admitted to a London hospital and subsequently to New York hospitals; perhaps one can call them *Intercontinental Munchausens*! Worse is the syndrome called Munchausen by proxy in which a parent, typically a mother, makes her child sick, gets the child admitted to the hospital, and gets the child to go through a lot of tests and treatment.

The syndrome is often difficult to manage, and these patients need a lot of psychological treatment, behavioral counseling, and strong family support.[7]

---

[7] January 2002

CHAPTER 8

Prescribing Hope

Empathy and open communication should be in your doctor's bag when treating seriously ill patients.

How would you react if your doctor told you that you have only six months to live? An impending death! Shock, depression, extreme anxiety, fear, despondency, and finally, "Oh what the heck, I have to die one day" attitude may ensue.

Ted Nolin (all names have been changed) felt this way when he was told that his days were numbered. At age seventy, heart failure was diagnosed. Ted had suffered from hypertension and diabetes, but when he was admitted a third time in severe pulmonary edema, gasping for breath, he thought that his worst fears were coming true. And his cardiologist, Dr. Hamby, wasn't very encouraging.

"Your husband has severe recurrent heart failure and probably has about six months to live," he told Mrs. Nolin. She was in tears. When the news was communicated to Ted, he was sad but stoic.

"It's God's will, I suppose," he said.

When Ted was admitted to the hospital for the fourth time, I happened to be on call for cardiology. The primary care physician called me and said, "Dr. Nathan, can you take care of this patient? He has dilated cardiomyopathy and recurrent heart failure, and Dr. Hamby thinks it is end-stage, and that he probably has only six more months. The patient and family know this. And Dr. Hamby is not coming to this hospital that often."

I knew Dr. Hamby still came to the hospital to take care of his private patients there. Thus, it appeared as if he had given up on Ted. Initially, I felt uncomfortable accepting the care of a dying patient just because his own cardiologist had given up on him.

"What do you want me to do? If his condition is end stage and everything has been done already, what more can I do except give comfort measures?" I politely asked the primary care physician. Finally, I accepted the patient and got ready to give some palliative care.

When I take over a patient's care from another physician it is always my policy to take a fresh history and review all aspects of the care to get true insight into his or her illness and see whether I can do anything more for the patient or find something that was overlooked. I want to learn the facts firsthand. All of us have busy schedules, and sometimes we just don't have enough time to sit down with the family and go over every aspect of disease management, despite our best efforts.

In reviewing the history, clinical data, and all the tests, it was apparent that the patient was indeed in end-stage heart failure. His work-up revealed that he had developed severe nonischemic dilated cardiomyopathy (enlarged flabby heart with an ejection fraction barely over 10 percent, normal being over 55 percent)—no doubt contributed in part by his diabetes, moderate hypertension, and some alcohol usage. He had been prescribed the standard drugs such as digoxin, diuretics, and vasodilators; however, the use of those drugs wasn't enough to prevent these recurrent admissions. Cardiac transplantation was considered, but Ted was too old for such exotic therapy.

Now that his care had been transferred to me, I decided to do the best I could to alleviate his suffering. When I saw him first in the emergency room, he was almost frozen with terror and had difficulty breathing, coupled with a sense of impending doom. I quickly got him out of his pulmonary edema. Once his condition was stable, I sat down with him and his wife to offer some counseling.

First, I discussed his diet, explaining how he could live without much salt, and I enforced some fluid restriction. "Only about six glasses of fluid total," I warned him.

"And one more thing," I added. "You can't simply sit at home and watch TV, waiting for death to come and grab you. Nobody in the world can make any predictions. But maybe we can beat death at its own game. What do you say?"

He must have thought that however provocative the idea might be, it was still a mostly hypothetical concept.

"How long one lives or when one is likely to die is a guessing game, and every individual is different. We must give it all we have before accepting defeat," I tried to encourage him.

Suddenly, his ears perked up. He became more attentive; there was a twinkle in his eyes now that I had never noticed before.

"You mean I have a chance?" he asked.

"Of course. Nothing is written in stone here. Together, we can stretch this heart to work a few more months or even years. Count your blessings, Ted. At least you don't have a rapidly spreading cancer."

The look on his face told me that he had changed from a timid man to an intrepid soldier ready to fight for his life.

"That's the spirit! Let's give it our best shot," I reassured him, knowing well that this journey would be difficult.

During the next several office visits, I started him on a gentle exercise program suitable for heart failure patients, and he even went to the hospital cardiac rehab program tailored to his needs. A home health care agency set up oxygen and administered occasional intravenous furosemide as needed. Although he was only mildly overweight, he managed to lose a few pounds.

Next, I went to work on his drug therapy. He was prescribed some of the newer medications such as carvedilol, which had only just come to the market at that time, a diuretic, potassium supplements, amiodarone for his ventricular arrhythmias, ace inhibitors, and later a dual-chamber pacemaker when he nearly coded one day with a slow heart rate. Finally, he started walking short distances without dyspnea. As he continued to improve, hospitalizations became less frequent, and his quality of life got better.

When he passed the much-anticipated first-year mark, both Ted and his family were exhilarated and brought me a nice card.

"So, it looks like I am going to make it, eh?" he asked my office staff with a smile.

It is often quoted in United States that heart failure is the single most frequent cause of hospitalization in older people and that the death rate from heart failure exceeds all forms of cancers combined. When not treated and monitored very carefully, heart failure progresses inexorably, shortening the ultimate life expectancy. Therefore, it is important to teach patients (and their relatives) how to take good care of themselves, follow a strict regimen of treatment, and modify lifestyles. The new treatments certainly have helped halt the progression of the disease and in some cases even reverse it.

As scientists, physicians generally put much emphasis on the technologic data of a patient while trying to gauge the prognosis. But medicine is also an art, and many other factors must be considered. The attending physician's words and body language are important when communicating with seriously ill patients. Along with the body, the mind also has boundless potential, and when used properly, can aid in the healing process. We must find time to dispense compassion, sympathy, and understanding when treating seriously ill patients. Instead of saying, "You have only six months to live," a better statement would be, "You have a serious illness, but we will do everything possible to control your illness and make you feel better." None of us can predict the future.

Ted Nolin lived for five more years and, finally, when I turned him over to hospice, his wife sent me a sweet note: "Thanks for giving Ted the hope he badly needed and then making all this happen. God bless."

Ted's case reconfirmed the general dictum: "Always give hope to your patients, and never let anybody take it away from them." As physicians, we must realize how much hope can bring to our patients by providing empathy, communicating openly, and acting in their best interests.[8]

---

[8] Reprinted with permission from *Medical Economics*: December 17, 2010 87: 24, pg 36–39. *Medical Economics* is a copyrighted publication of Advanstar Communications, Inc. All rights reserved.

CHAPTER 9

What Was Wrong
with My Patient?

It took a nurse's bedside observation to help me solve this medical mystery.

When I first saw sixty-five-year-old Patrick, he seemed very ill. At five feet ten inches and 137 pounds, he was gaunt and practically skin and bones. Thoughts of cancer, uncontrolled diabetes, and thyrotoxicosis raced through my mind. I wondered why he had waited so long to seek medical care.

Patrick was hearing-impaired, and I had difficulty getting a medical history. He turned up the volume on his hearing aid, but I still had to shout. Apparently he had come to my cardiac clinic because he'd been experiencing heartburn during his morning walks. Asked why he was so thin, he simply shrugged and said, "Oh, I've been underweight for some time now. I guess that's the way my body is."

Patrick's wife had passed away nearly three years before, but he looked happy and was at times garrulous. If he had any sadness, he internalized it well. He didn't have much help with cooking and cleaning. "TV dinners are my friends now," he said. "I don't know what I'd do without them."

The physical exam was unrevealing, except that he was a bit dehydrated. The electrocardiogram was mildly abnormal with nonspecific changes that raised the possibility of ischemia, so I admitted Patrick to the telemetry unit for further workup. Initial blood tests and chest X-rays were within normal limits, but his exercise stress test with nuclear imaging suggested that he did indeed have coronary artery disease.

So I scheduled Patrick for a cardiac catheterization. My interventional colleague called from the cath lab and notified me of a 90 percent lesion in the left anterior descending artery that looked ideal for angioplasty. Since we didn't have cardiac surgical facilities, Patrick was transferred to the nearby regional heart center and underwent a successful angioplasty. He should be OK now, I thought with relief.

At his follow-up exam a month later, Patrick was symptom-free but still dehydrated. Moreover, he was ashen, fatigued, and down to 135 pounds. He had lost his appetite, he told me. I was sure there was an occult malignancy somewhere. So I readmitted him for another battery of tests. A repeat stress test was negative for myocardial ischemia. The consulting oncologist declared him free of cancer. His mild anemia was expected to correct itself with improved diet and iron supplements. Upper and lower endoscopies were unrevealing. When he was ready to be discharged, the dietitian sat him down and reviewed basic lessons in nutrition and healthy cooking.

One month later, Patrick was in the ER. This time, it was hematuria and renal colic. The urologist reported a small stone in the left ureter that would probably pass with fluids and diuretics. He had lost another two pounds. One of the nurses with experience in pediatrics said his diagnosis should be "failure to thrive."

The following morning Deanna, the night nurse, called me and said, "Dr. Nathan, I've observed Patrick during all his admissions, and I talked to him at length last night. He's been very lonely since his wife died. His only son hasn't kept in touch with him, and he has no friends in the neighborhood."

"Do you think he's depressed?" I asked.

"Very much so," Deanna answered. "He told me, 'Every afternoon, I sit in my patio chair and think about my wife and the sweet life we had. We retired to Florida to enjoy our golden years, but we were not so lucky.

I've been a good person all my…' Then his voice trailed off and there were tears in his eyes."

I started Patrick on antidepressants. A consulting psychiatrist diagnosed him with situational depression.

"You know," the psychiatrist said, "there is bereavement and depression, and we need to differentiate the two. Patrick is more than sad. He is clearly depressed."

The social worker arranged for Patrick to get hot meals daily from the local Meals on Wheels program. We encouraged him to participate in church activities. Nurtured by personal and social contacts, he became more energetic and started gaining weight. At his next checkup, he'd put on three pounds. Not a giant leap, but tangible progress nevertheless. When I saw Deanna, I told her, "Thanks to you, Patrick is a lot better now."

Sometimes we don't realize that external appearances can be deceptive. Aging, with all its attendant medical problems, financial concerns, and loss of spouse and cohorts, often leads to depression. But some depressed patients put on a mask. Unless you lift the mask, the Patricks among our practice will continually "fail to thrive."[9]

[9] Reprinted with permission from *Medical Economics*: November 21, 2003, 80:22 pg 55-56. *Medical Economics* is a copyrighted publication of Advanstar Communications, Inc. All rights reserved.

CHAPTER 10

Death Comes Calling!

Office employees are not just workhorses; they are human beings with their own set of problems that need attention.

Usually I am greeted by Julie, my secretary, with a hearty good morning and a great big smile on her lips, as I walk into the office every day. Together we welcome the new day with all the thrills and hazards waiting to happen in a doctor's office. And together we handle a number of problems in the office like patients who have little patience in the waiting room, emergency patients dropping in unannounced, calls from insurance companies who want more details on the length of stay for a hospitalized patient, and so on. But Julie managed all these and much more with a smile, and I always trusted her judgment. But today she appeared to be a little glum.

"What is bothering you, Julie? You are not feeling well?"

"You know my father is visiting with me from New York. He is having headaches. He never had any headaches before. So I am very concerned. What could it be?"

"Well, why don't you bring him to the office? Let us check him out. Maybe it is nothing serious. Who doesn't get headaches these days? Living has become so stressful." I tried to lighten up the situation.

"Lately he is behaving like a child. He wants me at his side all the time. The moment I leave his room, he will call me for something. I don't know what to do."

I could see that Julie was a little disturbed. Apparently Frank had always been in good health, of hearty Italian stock, and at age seventy-eight, he still retained youthful looks and a cheery disposition. It was unusual for him to complain of anything. I could sense that there were mood changes too in Frank. This could be serious, I thought.

"Yesterday I found him crying when the headaches hit him. That really upset me. He never does that."

Soon our office became busy, and we plunged into work. I forgot all about Frank till the following morning when Julie called me with news. Frank had one of those splitting headaches again, and he was weeping uncontrollably. He was taken to the emergency room and got an elaborate workup. My associate saw him. A CAT scan of the brain was abnormal. It showed a distinct lesion about the size of a cherry, and the radiologist interpreted it as a tumor, arising from the frontal lobe. A neurologist was called in, and he confirmed the diagnosis. He said Julie's father would need surgery and should be transferred to St. Joseph's Hospital in Tampa for surgery. Julie wasn't happy about a transfer, since Tampa is at least fifty miles away from our rural Brooksville.

Now the insurance company came into the picture. Frank was enrolled with an HMO that wanted him to be transferred only to Tampa General Hospital, the approved hospital. So Julie had no choice and within a few hours Frank was in the ambulance heading toward Tampa General Hospital. Julie didn't mind being forced to choose a different hospital. It was the suddenness and the gravity of the situation that bothered her. She was really devastated. Her father came down here from New York to escape the harsh winter and spend some time with his favorite daughter. Now he had to endure a major surgery, a brain surgery, nothing less. He was facing life's worst winter with all its fury.

There were more tests at Tampa General, including an MRI that confirmed that Frank's was no ordinary headache. Julie called my home and gave my wife all the little details. My wife, a pediatrician and office manager of our office, and Julie had always been good friends. Between them they avoided patient complaints and made sure the office was run well. Julie told my wife how the surgeon pointed out the images of the brain, which clearly showed the ugly tumor with tentacles all around viciously attacking rest of the brain. The tumor was clearly malignant and treatment options were few, the only one being immediate brain surgery.

Frank underwent excision of the tumor the following morning. It was very exhausting for everybody involved. The surgery lasted for nearly five and a half hours. For Julie it looked like this surgery would never be over. They took out a large tumor, the size of a lemon, from the frontal lobe. All was well at the end of surgery. Hopefully the recovery process has started, she thought.

But after twenty-four hours, Frank still hadn't woken up. Julie was concerned, and I was too. Although brain surgery is more complicated than others, he should have been opening his eyes by this time. I eagerly awaited the telephone call from Tampa General Hospital. It took almost thirty-six hours for Frank to open his eyes. He was still confused and dazed. The neurosurgeon assured Julie that this was not unusual; after all, this was brain surgery, nothing less.

But Julie couldn't bear to look at her father the way he was lying in the intensive care unit connected to a respirator with an intravenous feeding tube, a tube through the nose into his stomach, so many monitors going at the same time, and most of them making weird sounds. Till a few days ago he was such a feisty, vibrant guy, cracking jokes and loving life. Now he was close to death. What an irony.

Brain surgery can be very tricky. Often it takes long hours to meticulously isolate the tumor and cut it out. Paralysis of one side can occur as a complication of the surgery especially if you cut out more tissue. It can result in scars in the brain leading to seizures. We didn't know what to expect after this complicated surgery.

We eagerly awaited the pathology results. We hoped against hope that this would be a benign tumor. But I knew in my heart that this had to be a malignant tumor. When I questioned Julie again, she said that Frank developed the headaches just about a month prior to surgery. So this had to be a rapidly growing lesion, in medical terms. And unfortunately, that is the way it turned out. The surgeon informed her it was an aggressive cancer, called glioblastoma, and would need additional radiotherapy.

"Do people recover from this kind of cancer ever?" Julie wanted to know. I had to hedge the answer. "There is no telling, Julie, what with all these wonderful new treatments. Cures for many cancers are being reported almost on a daily basis." Although the diagnosis entailed bad prognosis I didn't want to crush her hope.

"That is good to know." She seemed to be satisfied with the answer, at least for now.

Frank's recovery from surgery was slow but by the end of first week he managed to walk with a walker, speak a few words, and relearn all those processes that we take for granted. He was able to take a liquid diet, and intravenous feeding tubes were removed. Julie let out a big sigh of relief; one crisis is over. Death had come calling, but for now it would have to wait. This surgery was successful.

Now we had to tell Frank that he had developed brain cancer. "How do you tactfully tell a person that his headaches are from a cancer?" Julie asked me. I didn't have any answer. But Frank had to be told the truth. And he was initially very discouraged after he heard the verdict. He didn't ask the traditional question: "Why me?" Instead he accepted the diagnosis with grace and courage. An old Italian trooper with a great zest for life, Frank wanted to be well at any cost. And I could sense that he was not going to sit around and feel sorry for himself. He wasn't scared.

The diagnosis of cancer heralds a long complicated process with many vicissitudes. It is a death sentence for most people. Now, Frank needed radiotherapy. A full course of radiation will last about a month and it can often be complicated with nausea, fatigue, and pain. It is not a simple process by any means.

Poor Julie! She had to juggle with all the chores in the house and then run to the hospital to attend to her father. Her youngest child was still in school and needed some attention. Fortunately her husband was very understanding and pitched in. Amid all this, she also managed to put in a few hours at the office. She was worried about my office running smoothly in her absence. I used to compare Julie to the Indian goddess Lakshmi with four arms; she could do many jobs simultaneously with ease. Phones rang off the wall, irate patients wanted to see the doctor right away, drug representatives walked in and tried to chat her up to gain entry to see the doctor, and so on. She was the best multitasking human machine, I'd ever seen.

Julie frequently gave me a progress report of her dad. As always I was ready with my free advice and comfort, which she seemed to appreciate. Julie literally became the private nurse for her father and chauffeur for the household, especially taking him to the radiation center and back, doctor's office, and much more. Whenever possible she sat at his bedside and even held his hand when he slept. She talked to him even when he was confused. She cradled him when he was in the grips of a headache.

Interestingly Julie never missed a day at the office. I never realized how my elderly patients and their relatives coped with when one was struck with a serious deadly illness. Frank now needed total care and their HMO plan would not allow a home health nurse to come daily. Once the radiation therapy was completed, the oncologist couldn't do anything more. My associate and I acted as the family physicians for her father.

Julie was the doting daughter while Frank was teetering in and out of his lucid intervals. Often he would call for her and became very upset when she left for the office. Sometimes he would forget her name and call her by another name. This would elicit tears in her eyes. Her mother was a nervous wreck throughout this ordeal.

As expected Frank started deteriorating and slipped into a coma. I asked Julie to go and sit with her father as long as she wanted, and she was glad to get two days off. Finally, with all his children at his bedside Frank said good-bye to the world. For a while Julie was inconsolable but finally recovered.

The funeral was well attended with many of our patients and their spouses joining in to give condolences. Julie had regained a measure of her composure by this time. She was so popular among our patients and in the office, it was not surprising that everybody rallied around her. After a week, she returned to work seemingly recovered from the ordeal. All of us were happy to see Julie back to work.

Now I don't look at my employees as workhorses, but simply as human beings just like me with their own set of problems and crises in life. I also learned how to get involved in their lives and produce a positive effect. I knew sooner or later I could be in the same position as well with older people living in my house and me not getting any younger.[10]

[10] February 1998

CHAPTER 11

Never Too Old!

The first day of joining the teaching medical center as an attending physician, turned out to be a learning experience for the author.

July 1976

I was a young medical attending doing teaching rounds in Jersey City Medical Center in New Jersey. Having just finished my cardiovascular fellowship training I was eager to prove myself in front of the bright young interns and residents. Perhaps even win the best teaching attending award during the year-end residents' party.

"Who is presenting the first case?" I asked with a touch of authority.

"I guess I will go first," said a timid intern reluctantly; he had recently arrived from Philippines. Having been up all night admitting patients and attending to emergencies, he appeared a bit weary and diffident. Maybe I can teach him a thing or two today, I told myself.

"This seventy-two-year-old woman, a widow who lives by herself, presented to the ER with mild fever, pain, and swelling of the right knee," he started. I asked the rest of the audience, the differential diagnosis before any laboratory data were spelled out.

"Gout" somebody in the audience announced with confidence.

"Possible, what else?" I asked.

"Chondrocalcinosis."

"Maybe, but does it present with fever?" I prodded

"Monoarticular rheumatoid arthritis."

"Very good, especially in a woman. Let us have a few more, guys," I encouraged them.

"How about septic arthritis?" the intern presenting the case suggested tentatively.

"Yes, that is a possibility but...is there a source?" I inquired.

"None visible; no trauma or knee surgery, no systemic infection. No history of venereal infections."

"So..." I raised my eyebrows in partial disapproval. "OK, let us have some lab data now. Did you get any synovial fluid?"

The intern gave me some lab data. The CBC showed the white cell count was increased. Joint aspiration was only partially successful, yielding a small amount of fluid. No uric acid crystals to suggest gout were seen, but there were plenty of white cells indicating possible a septic arthritis. So far nothing was growing in the blood or synovial fluid cultures.

"So, what could it be? It looks like this case is a puzzle!" I tentatively suggested. Suddenly the authority in my voice started fading. The young intern felt that we should treat this woman for septic arthritis, for now. We had some more didactic discussions, analyzed the case in detail, and decided that there was no clear diagnosis at this time; we would have to wait for the labs. The whole entourage then marched on to the cafeteria for the lunch break.

That afternoon I came back to the same floor to do an urgent consult. The intern hadn't left the floor, and as soon as he saw me he came over smiling and announced that he had a working diagnosis on the morning's case.

"So what did the cultures show?" I was confident the lab had come to our rescue.

"Cultures are not available yet. But I came back and got a better history."

"Oh, what is it?" I was eager to know the new facts.

It turned out that this old woman took in a young boarder, about twenty-eight years old. He would snuggle up with her during the cold nights. She obviously didn't object. And indeed the vaginal examination revealed a slightly purulent discharge with diplococci on gram stain. Needless to say, that the cultures from the discharge grew gonococci, the bacteria responsible for the venereal disease called gonorrhea.

When the intern confronted the woman with regard to her indiscretion, she had this much to say: "What could I do? I didn't want to lose my tenant, you know."

"At least you don't have to worry about getting pregnant." The intern tried to lighten up the situation.

So, my first day in this teaching hospital turned out to be a true learning experience. I guess you are never too old![11]

---

[11] First published in *Cortlandt Forum*: November 1999, 12:11, pg 99.

CHAPTER 12

Humor to Reduce Practice Stress?

Physicians can use humor to entertain their patients. Patients often use humor to get your attention or as an outlet for their emotions and frustrations.

Lately, our profession has been besieged by too many conflicts and up-heavals. The stress level is at an all-time high. The physician-patient relationship has suffered considerably. My good friend, Michael Rosenberg, an orthopedic surgeon in his young fifties, announced during lunch time one day that he is quitting.

"Why, at such a young age?" I asked.

"Oh, it has become too dangerous to practice now. You don't need much to be hit with a malpractice suit these days."

I guess this is the prevailing sentiment with many others too. The escalating premiums for liability insurance, the ferocious malpractice climate, the tight stranglehold of bureaucracy, P4P (pay for performance) reform, the latest entry into these conundrums, and more have gotten us all stumped. I know many others are also considering early exit strategies. Michael is a concert pianist too, trained at the famous Juilliard, so he can quit. But that is certainly not an option for me or for many others except for those who are in their sixties and truly ready for retirement.

Unfortunately it is not just the medical profession; life itself is full of chaos and conflicts these days. So what we need to do is put some fun and humor into our practice. After all, our patients have entrusted us with their lives. That is a great honor and privilege.

Laughter is still one of the best medicines that I know of and laughing with others—especially a good belly laugh—can be a powerful antidote to stress. In addition it can be a very good coping mechanism against life's multitudes of stresses and stressors. All of us will agree that developing a good sense of humor is no laughing matter either.

Once I started lightening up and listening to my patients' stories, life and my practice became more enjoyable. As Hippocrates advised, physicians should cultivate a serious and respectable image but at the same time use wit in interacting with their patients. Now humor is always on my radar screen. You would be surprised how patients open up and entertain you with interesting snippets from their lives—some of them quite hilarious and others very poignant. All you need to do is just be patient and listen to their stories. Let me give you a sampler.

Vernon

Vernon, a big, burly man, suffered from hypertension and peripheral vascular disease; but he continued to imbibe moderately in spite of my constant advice against it. He came to the office one day with angina but wanted me to take a look at the blister on his foot that had just broken and was hurting him a bit. My nurse cleaned his foot with an alcohol wipe, and it burned him quite a bit.

"Oh, boy, that alcohol stings a lot," he complained semi-jokingly.

"Oh, Vernon, don't be a baby now," I teased him.

After applying the dressing, I prescribed an antibiotic cream and told him "Clean it twice a day with alcohol wipe and apply the cream."

"You think I can apply the alcohol from inside?" he asked with mock seriousness. We had a good laugh.

Chris

The story of Christopher is quite interesting. Although only forty years old, Chris initially presented to the ER with palpitations from paroxysmal supraventricular tachycardia. His heart rate was close to 200/minute when he arrived but converted quickly to regular sinus rhythm with simple treatment. Subsequent tests were negative for any major underlying cardiac problem.

When I inquired about his alcohol usage, Janet, his wife, quickly obliged: "Doc, he has two to three cocktails a day with his buddies and sometimes more. He says he is planning to quit!" After taking a detailed history, I sensed that he was suffering from alcohol-related arrhythmias. I advised him to stop drinking. "An occasional glass of red wine is OK," I added not to disappoint him completely.

He quit his booze and his palpitations subsided dramatically. Then he stopped coming to the office. One day, somewhat unexpectedly, Janet brought him to the office again. "Doc, his palpitations have started again," she said.

"That is interesting. He was OK for a while though. How come?"

"You shouldn't have talked to him about wine."

"Why, what is the matter? I thought I gave you good advice." I was a bit surprised.

"As soon as he gets back home from the office he fills six tall glasses with wine, and then he sips them slowly all evening. And he tells everybody that Dr. Nathan has recommended that wine is good for the heart!"

"No wonder his heart is acting up again," I said.

I was bemused at the misinterpretation of my advice and the surprising turn of events but apologized anyway for not being very clear with my instructions. Patients always interpret your advice the way it suits them. And then they try to convince you that that's what you told them in the first place. After some gentle scolding and repeat advice, he stopped alcohol usage completely and was once again better. This also taught me to be careful with what I say and how I say it.

Priscilla

Priscilla is a true bleached blond. She gave me a real surprise during her initial visit. I admired her hair, and seeing my looks she said seriously, "I am very light-headed."

Thinking she is dizzy, I asked her to lie down quickly and started taking her pulse. Then, with a big grin, she said: "Oh, I simply meant I am a blond!"

"You frightened me a little," I said jokingly. We had a good laugh together.

Phillip

Phillip, one of our elderly patients, had a recent retinal surgery. He drove to my office for his cardiac checkup. When my nurse, Rosie, asked him to step onto the scales, he missed the platform and almost fell.

"Phil, can you see well?" Rosie asked

"Rosie, I can't see a thing. I just had the retinal surgery, you know."

"Really, then how can you drive?"

"Not well, but the Lord will take care of me."

"Mm…How about others on the road, Phil?" Rosie asked.

Reggie

Reggie's case was of course different—rather poignant. He has been quite obese all his life, and because of his coronary heart disease and mild heart failure I have been constantly on his back to lose weight.

One day he was diagnosed with lung cancer and soon developed multiple metastases in many organs. As expected he lost quite a bit of weight. On his latest visit he said as if jokingly, "Well, finally I have lost weight as you had asked me to, Dr. Nathan…" His voice trailed off.

I tried hard to hide the teardrops welling in my eyes.

Now humor is spilling into my other activities too. In our Yoga for Relaxation class on Wednesday evenings, there are at least four doctors present at any given time. We keep our beepers in one corner, stretch the yoga mats, and get started. One day our beepers started going off one by one, and all of us had to get up and go and look at the messages every time to see if it was urgent. All the beepers had the same tone!

"There goes our relaxation session," commented the benevolent instructor.

Physicians can use humor to entertain their patients. Patients often use humor to get your attention or as an outlet for their emotions and frustrations. In these days, primary care physicians are working harder, seeing more volume with less income, and specialists are under pressure because they have to cover so many hospitals and their schedule is tight. Hence, it is difficult to spend quality time with each patient. A little attentiveness to a patient's stories, a touch of humor in your conversation, and a pat on the back usually puts a smile on a patient's face and improves his or her will to survive.

As Norman Cousins says in his famous book *Anatomy of An Illness*, "…it helps make it possible for good things to happen." It will also make your day go easier. This is why "laughter, especially a good belly laughter, is considered the best medicine."[12]

---

[12] An abbreviated version was published in the *Journal of the Florida Medical Association*, Pg 10–12, July 2004.

CHAPTER 13

A Breach of Trust

A novice to the practice, I was taken for a ride by a codeine addict. So beware of these pitfalls.

I eased up a little on the gas pedal as I came upon the sign, "Welcome to Brooksville." So this would be the little town I will practice for the rest of my life. Finally I am out of the dull, dreary rat race of New York City with its really cold winters. The morning ray of Florida sunshine encouraged my spirits. I rolled the window down and let the sights and sounds of the new town come in. Two old men were leisurely chatting in the local gas station.

The senior physician who recruited me was full of enthusiasm and optimism. Most patients were either retirees or farmers who paid their bills on time and didn't give any trouble. That was what I wanted to hear. My dream was to build a large practice.

The first day at the office was exciting but still pretty uneventful: just half a dozen patients with mostly not-so-serious chest pains and a few coughs and colds. Standard fare for an internist/ cardiologist's office. All had good insurance too, unlike the ones I used to see in our cardiology clinic at my previous medical center in New Jersey.

That night, I got a call from the answering service. "Ray," a twenty-nine-year-old gentleman, recently moved from Atlanta, had a severe, almost incessant cough and needed some quick remedy. Apparently I was recommended to him by a Dr. Patel. Patel is such a common last name among North Indians and there are many who have settled in the US, and I wouldn't know who this particular Patel was unless I had at least his or her first name. The gentleman specifically wanted only "Tussionex," the most potent codeine-containing narcotic cough syrup. Being a novice to private practice, I didn't quite know the importance of this "controlled substance." Anyway, he hadn't established with my practice. So I asked him to either go to the ER or come to my office first thing in the morning.

Ray was already pacing up and down, restless and anxious, by the time I got to the office. The nurse came running in and whispered in my ear that this new patient pretended to be some dignitary and was here on a short vacation. Apparently I had been highly recommended to him. I liked to believe his story, but I wasn't sure if he was putting me on. Could I have already become so famous here? I didn't think so, but I wasn't going to argue that. He had been coughing incessantly and had had a complete workup in a large general hospital in Atlanta. Only a certain cough syrup, Tussionex, would relieve his pain, he said. He wanted a prescription. I offered to do some tests to get to the bottom of his problem, at least to reevaluate the current status. Many things in medicine change quickly and frequently, I reminded him. He seemed to be reluctant to have even a cursory examination, saying that all these had been done elsewhere.

I was a little confused and really didn't know what the next course of action should be. I certainly wanted to keep him as my patient and do what was necessary to relieve his cough, and yet I didn't want to accede to his demands so quickly. He would think I was a pushover and his demands would only escalate in the future. Anyway, this time, I gave him a prescription for a 12 oz. of Tussionex and told him this should last him for at least a week, and if he didn't improve he would need further tests. He thanked me profusely and promptly paid his charges.

Three days later, I got a call from the local pharmacist for a refill for Ray. What? Had he already finished his one week's quota in just three days? I wanted to see him in the office, and he reluctantly came in with all kinds of excuses. He was in agony and had to take more.

"You are my only doctor here, and I need more medicine just to keep my sanity. It is your duty to give this to me," he said a little emphatically. There was perhaps a hint of a threat in his words. This time, I was the bold guy and didn't want to oblige that quickly. Also, how could I keep giving a patient, whom I hardly knew, a codeine-containing cough syrup?

My antennae went up. I called the previous hospital in Atlanta, where he said he had full workup. But there were no records. Same result with many other hospitals in the area. So I knew the whole story was a fake. I confronted Ray with this new information, and he became visibly irate, said a few expletives, and stomped out of the office. A few minutes later, I got a call from the local pharmacist again, asking for a refill for Ray, who had approached him with my prescription.

"You are new here, Doc?" the benevolent pharmacist asked me knowingly as he introduced himself.

"Yes, I started practice only the other day. Why do you ask?"

"It is about this prescription for Ray," he answered.

"Oh, I don't want to give any more Tussionex to the gentleman," I told the pharmacist.

"I agree, you shouldn't. You don't know what kind of guys you run into, these days," he cautioned me. "Everybody wants a euphoric pill or elixir these days and the new doctor often becomes the target," he added for good measure. There was good advice in his words.

Clearly I was being taken for a ride. I knew I could easily fall into the trap, if I didn't watch out, as much as I wanted to build a large practice. I wondered how many doctors he had abused in the past.

For a moment my introspection got the better of me. Why this facade? What was wrong with him? Was he perhaps a narcotic addict? Questions, questions, but no answers. The pharmacist shared my suspicions that Ray might be canvassing yet another doctor in order to support his Tussionex habit. Clearly he was addicted to codeine. At any rate, he never showed up in the office again, but I did make a critical remark in his chart for posterity.[13]

---

[13] First published as a condensed version in *Cortlandt Forum* 1995 8: 6, pg 55.

CHAPTER 14

The Last Stop!

"Oh, please, never get old!" said Margaret, the author's neighbor, one day.

For nearly two years now, Room 328 has been her home. It is a small room she shares with another woman about her age. A curtain in the middle keeps her privacy. Sometimes she remembers her name, sometimes not. She needs help with bathing and needs a wheelchair to get around. She has lost a lot of weight. But when I asked her about her son, the wrinkled face instantly lit up. "Oh, Peter is fine. He is building a house in Mexico." Suddenly she seems to be regaining her memory.

That is Margaret, my neighbor for the past fifteen years.

When we moved to this quiet neighborhood in Brooksville, blessed with southern country charm, the first persons we met were Margaret and her husband, Joe. They were in their sixties. Margaret had an inquisitive mind and a sharp intellect to match that. She wanted to know all about India, since I told her that my wife and I hailed from that subcontinent. Their house was neat with well-kept grounds, a veritable paradise every spring, full of blooming azaleas, camellias, and gardenias. Those who passed by the house would often stop to admire the flowers.

One winter, when they returned from their annual northern summer trip, I didn't see Joe. "Oh, Joe passed on while we were up in Boston. You know he had chronic lung problems, he was a chemist all his life, and maybe that is why."

Margaret had clearly aged after this trip. "Stress has taken its toll," I told myself. Soon Margaret became my patient as she developed one illness after another. Initially it was her heart, needing a valve replacement. Then her gallbladder had to come out. After each operation, she had to go to a nursing home for convalescence, which she hated with a passion. Her only son, Peter, was always away, constantly changing jobs and traveling.

Slowly Margaret's health deteriorated even further. First it was a mini-stroke, then heart failure. Once she fainted in her house. When she came to her senses, the only telephone number she could remember was mine. That was my first house call after I arrived in this town. With a pacemaker, the dizziness cleared, and her energy returned.

Spunky and independent, the merry widow would often embark on shopping trips, driving her old model Ford at 5 mph on our 35 mph street. Oh, how she loved life and everything around her, especially the big house on two and a half acres! Occasionally, Tom, her grandson, would drop by and on those days she would be beaming, bragging proudly about him.

But the mini-strokes never relented, and she became quite frail. It had become clear that she couldn't live by herself, so the son made the decision for her. Margaret must go to a nursing home…permanently. That day I agonized about her. How desperately she wanted to live in her own house!

A few months later, on a glorious autumn Sunday, my wife and I paid a visit to Brooksville Manor, a popular local nursing home. Most of the residents were cheerful, others lost in their own foggy world. As I walked past them, their eyes seemingly following me, I made my mental diagnoses: strokes, Alzheimer's, Parkinsonism…

Margaret was in her room, finishing her lunch. I gently held her hand and asked: "Do you remember me?"

"Well, your voice is familiar. But I can't place you."

"I am your neighbor. My house is just across yours on Cindy Drive."

"Let my neighbors go to hell! What do they care? I don't remember anybody." And pointing to her tray, she yelled, "Where is my milk? They always forget to bring my milk."

What a change! I felt sad and disappointed. She had already forgotten me, her neighbor, her family physician, and cardiologist. Today, she seemed reticent, irate, and clearly depressed. This was not the friendly neighbor whom I once knew.

I gently started talking about her house, her son, and the grandson, whom she adored. Then I introduced myself again.

Suddenly, everything seemed to come back to her.

"Now I remember you, Doctor, *how are you?*" And turning toward my wife, she asked, "*And who are you?*"

"I am Susheela, Mrs. Nathan."

"Oh, yes. I remember you too."

"Your son and grandson visit you often?" I inquired gently.

"They're all too busy, you know. They come when they can, maybe once a year. But I can see them every day. Look!" She pointed to an old faded group photo of her entire family, on the night table.

I was at a loss for words.

"Oh, how I wish I could go back to my house and take care of my plants! Are they still there?" she asked earnestly.

"Oh, your house is in fine shape, don't worry. The plants too," I said encouragingly, knowing that no one was tending to them. "It will be there whenever you come back."

She didn't answer. A couple of tears welled up in her eyes. A little pause, then she sighed. "This is my home now. These girls here are very nice to me. With my poor health, how can I live in my house alone?"

Then as an afterthought, she said: "If only I could go home and stay there for one more day! That is my only dream now."

My eyes also became teary. I wanted to gently remind her that "dreams come with their own expiration dates," a line I had heard somewhere before.

After a pause, she said, squinting her eyes, "How I wish I could see you good! After my last stroke and then the cataract, I am virtually blind."

Suddenly I had a lump in my throat.

I saw the shattered heart of an old woman stuck in a nursing home, where she was withering away in loneliness. Once she was a lovely daughter, then a passionate wife, later a caring mother, and finally a doting grandmother. Now she had no more roles to play.

Past memories flooded my mind. Our bucolic neighborhood full of live oaks and Spanish moss, pines, and flower-laden bushes. Deer sauntering in the backyards, munching on our precious hibiscus and roses without a care. Peacocks showing off their plumes and dancing on cloudy days. Possums with eternally frightened looks crossing the street at night. Armadillos digging up the lawns, looking for insects to eat. Raccoons pilfering the trash cans. Every morning the neighborhood wakes up to the sound track of an Audubon orchestra. Margaret and I had been very much part of that scenery for the past decade and half. And now she knew she could never go back to her private little paradise.

I suddenly asked her: "Do you want to come with us for a walk?"

"Oh, Doctor, I have no legs. How can I walk?"

I cast one fleeting glance at her wasted legs. Tears welled up in my eyes.

After saying good-bye, I stepped out and looked around. There were a few people sitting in wheelchairs like zombies. One couple was walking along the corridor, as though they had just learned how to walk. An old woman, well dressed with her handbag and all, was harassing the ward clerk, repeating constantly, "I want to go home, call a cab… now!"

A sad world indeed. I think Margaret was right, when she told me before she came to the nursing home, "Oh, please, never get old."[14]

---

[14] First published in the *Journal of the Florida Medical Association*, October, 2002, pg 20.

CHAPTER 15

Faith Healing

Faith and science have always respected each other's territory. But can faith override scientific reasoning and evidence-based management?

The year, I believe, was 1979. I was then the acting chief of cardiology at Jersey City Medical Center in New Jersey.

When my secretary announced that there were two saffron-robed ladies with flowing hair and *tilak** on their foreheads, looking for me, I knew they must be from the Holy Hindu Order of Stroudsburg, Pennsylvania. Last summer, I had taken my ten-year-old son for the Hindu Heritage Camp at the temple premises and had become acquainted with both the Divine Mother, who was the head priestess, although a Jew by birth, and her first assistant, Swami Devi. We shared the same religious beliefs. The idyllic setting and the serene atmosphere of the temple really captured my imagination. Women, who dominated the priesthood there, were conducting the temple activities remarkably well.

They must be here for some donation, I said to myself. These religious orders depend solely on public support. Their unexpected appearance in the corridors of this busy medical institution must have evoked a lot of curiosity. "*Could this be another one of those cults?*" they must have wondered.

But it was the duo from Pennsylvania, for sure. I exchanged a few pleasantries. Then Swami Devi explained the purpose of the visit: "Lately

73

Divine Mother finds it difficult to climb the steps of the temple. She feels exhausted toward the end of the day. So we came to consult the only cardiologist we knew."

"Oh, I feel flattered," I said blushing. "But you didn't have to travel all the way to Jersey City. I could have arranged for you to be seen by a local cardiologist," I added in a sympathetic tone.

"Well, we really wanted to see you, so here we are," said Swami Devi.

I completed a full physical examination on the divine mother and took an electrocardiogram. The diagnosis was obvious. She had typical mitral stenosis—narrowing of the valve between left atrium and left ventricle—which had led to congestive heart failure. My technician obliged me with a quick echocardiogram that confirmed the diagnosis of severe calcific mitral stenosis (narrowing of the mitral valve on the left side of the heart), dilated left atrium and all the other features of advanced disease.

"Divine Mother, you have a heart condition that has resulted in blockage of a valve, and it is not letting through enough blood. This is causing congestion of the lungs. That is why you feel so exhausted and short of breath," the scientist in me tried to explain, without causing any panic in these simple folks. Then I outlined the treatment option, which of course consisted of a cardiac catheterization followed by cardiac surgery if the narrowing of the valve was severe enough. "Medicines alone will not be enough. And cardiac surgery has become easier to do now, and we don't see many complications," I added.

"Oh, no, that would be impossible," Swami Devi said softly.

"Why is that?" I was a little puzzled. "This shouldn't interrupt your schedule too much. Maybe ten days at the most, including the surgery."

"But, *she is the divine mother,*" reminded Swami Devi with an ethereal glance. That meant no further explanation was necessary.

All this time, the divine mother kept her stately posture with an amusing smile. She was in another world. She must have felt that she was different from others, the enlightened one.

During the next couple of minutes, we communicated mainly through our eyes. It was evident that the divine mother wasn't going to be submitted to any surgery done by a mere mortal. She obviously had greater faith in her religion and vocation and expected the whole process to cure by itself. Finally, they accepted a prescription from me for a couple of drugs that would relieve the fluid accumulation in the lungs and regulate the heartbeats, and they left with profuse thanks. They would call me for a follow-up if needed, they said.

I did not hear from them afterward.

The following year, I took my son again to the same Hindu Heritage Camp and briefly met the priestesses. Divine mother looked a little chubbier. We chatted for a while, mostly on Hindu philosophy. Although I wanted to know more about her health, she politely evaded the issue and was more content to talk about loftier things: the temple, upbringing of children, the achievements of the Holy Order, etc. *She was unquestionably the high priestess.* Everybody there worshipped her as if she were a goddess. And she seemed to enjoy her exalted position.

Three days later, I got a frantic call from my son.

"Daddy, come and get me right now." He sounded very agitated and perturbed.

"What is the matter, son? Don't you like it there anymore?"

"No, No...it's total chaos here...you ready for this?"

"Tell me, what is it?" The suspense was getting to me now.

"The divine mother suddenly passed away this morning!"

I was speechless.

Faith and science have always respected each other's territory. Yet, I wonder if a tragedy could have been averted...but then, who am I to make that judgment? I guess we shall always remain vulnerable to our convictions. While faith is considered as an adjunct in the healing process of almost any illness, it cannot override scientific reasoning and evidence-based management for serious diseases. As one of my good friends, an eminent cardiologist in Florida, says: "Faith can certainly help to heal, whether the ailment is physical, mental, or social—especially when used in the right dosage, for the right reasons, and in the right combination."

* *Tilak* (from Sanskrit) means decorative ornamental dot on the forehead, worn by Hindu ladies.[15]

[15] A condensed version was first published in *Cortlandt Forum*, June 25, 1997.

CHAPTER 16

An Unscheduled Stop *The Story of a Successful House Call*

The miracle of a dying man returning to life just with home treatment and without any fancy medicines! The author still doesn't know the reason for the patient's coma.

This happened shortly before I left India for the US in 1972. I was a practicing internist in a small metropolitan area in Kerala, my home state. The practice was quite busy and often my clients would come and knock on the door any time, irrespective of day or night. And in those days the consultation rooms were simply the front part of my house. That was the way it was for almost all private practitioners. I managed with just two rooms, one served as the waiting room, the other a consultation and examination room—all in one.

One afternoon while I was busy seeing a patient, there appeared to be a lot of commotion in the narrow road in front of my office. It looked like somebody was shouting directions to a driver...

"Turn a bit to the right, you are going to hit the wall, now back off a bit, now straighten the wheel..."

There were awful sounds of tires screeching on the rough surface of our poorly paved road. People were shouting,

"Can't you see the sign, man? No buses or trucks on this road, this is not a bus route, please. You will kill somebody," an irate pedestrian was admonishing the driver.

It turned out the driver was trying to negotiate a large passenger bus through this narrow road in front of my office. I wondered why, since the adjacent road about fifty feet away was much wider and designated as the regular bus route. He could have simply parked the bus there and walked to his destination, wherever it was in this small road.

Then I noted that he had just stopped his vehicle right in front of my gate. A well-dressed gentleman got out and came right to my consultation room. Although there were several ahead of him waiting to see me, he knocked on my examining room door. I gently opened and peeked outside to see who was in such a hurry.

"Sir, it is an emergency. We want to take you to our house to see my sick father. He is very ill, he may die soon," he said in a hurry. He appeared to be very anxious, and beads of sweat dotted his forehead.

Apparently his elderly father, Mr. P. Nair, a prominent businessman and the owner of a commercial bus service with a large fleet of buses, had taken ill suddenly. He would need urgent attention. They did not want to take him to the hospital or anyplace without being initially evaluated by a competent doctor.

"Why did you bring a bus? I can't travel in this one," I said somewhat jokingly. "Don't you have a car?"

"Yes, we do have two, but both of them are not available right at this moment. Hence we decided to bring this bus. It was there after the morning run. So we grabbed it to avoid any delay," he said somewhat apologetically. "Sorry for creating such a commotion here," he added.

House calls are quite common in India since many older persons dislike hospitalization even if it is a major emergency. And they think that people are hospitalized only for terminal conditions. Most of the village folks feel that the hospital is usually the last stop since many do not come back alive, at least in those days. Plus they all like to be treated in their own home environment.

I decided to travel in my own car and follow the bus. The scene at the patient's home was interesting if not puzzling. A lot of people had crowded in and around the house spilling into the large front yard and other areas his compound. All of them looked gloomy, as though witnessing an unfolding tragedy.

I entered the house with my doctor's bag, thinking that I may be too late. It turned out that Mr. Nair happened to be a seventy-two-year-old patriarch of an old aristocratic Hindu family. He was most likely developing a stroke and was already in a coma. His wife, several of his children, and a few cousins and friends had crowded around the bed, all very distraught and weeping. A traditional oil lamp was burning auspiciously at the head of the bed, the body covered with a white sheet except for the face, and flowers scattered at the foot of the bed...all symbolic of last rites in the Hindu religion. They didn't expect him to make it through the night.

First I took a detailed history and then examined him thoroughly. He had suffered from hypertension for some time and suddenly became unconscious. No history of diabetes mellitus. His pulse was a little weak, maybe even irregular, and blood pressure had dropped. He was in a deep coma, the limbs were flaccid, and breathing was slow and labored. The skin was a bit cool to touch. There was no fever or other signs of sepsis. He looked practically dead!

Obviously Mr. Nair had suffered a major stroke, I decided. The differential diagnosis was between a cerebral hemorrhage and subarachnoid hemorrhage. Both are very serious conditions with a poor prognosis. The patriarch's three sons were eagerly awaiting my opinion. So I told them: "Your father needs hospitalization for observation and intensive management. The outlook at this time is a bit grim."

"Oh, no, that is out of question," the oldest son, who acted as the spokesperson, said. The wife was too grief stricken to talk. "We don't want him to be dragged through the hospital and all these tests and poking the skin...We just want to make sure that good physician like you has seen him. He hates hospitals. We will just give him comfort measures till God makes His decision, one way or the other."

I got the impression that the family had already given up and was simply waiting for the final curtain to close on a well-lived life. Clearly they didn't want him to be hospitalized, nor did they want any aggressive workup or intensive care. CT scans of the brain were not available at that time. But they wanted me to do whatever I could do at home to keep him comfortable without pain or shortness of breath. And if there is any magic drug in my sleeves, that would be welcome too.

I made sure that he was not in a hypoglycemic coma. One of the local nurses was summoned to the house, and we started IV dextrose that would maintain adequate blood sugar levels, give him some nutrition, and also to keep a line open to administer any further drugs. I taught them how to clear the secretions accumulating in the mouth and to take care of the airways. They learned about seizure precautions. Then I gave a dose of IV Decadron (a steroid), an important initial treatment for strokes to be repeated every eight hours for the next two days. This should at least decrease the cerebral edema of the brain (swelling of the brain) and might improve the brain function.

I didn't expect him to survive either.

What happened subsequently can only be called dramatic and unbelievable. In the next few days the patient gradually woke up and started moving his limbs. Then he started taking medicines and food by mouth. Although the progress was slow it was steady, and eventually he was able to walk with support. The recovery was quite remarkable, nearly complete.

A few weeks afterward the family visited my house, this time in a car. Mr. Nair, now walking with a cane, also came along. He was beaming and thanked me profusely. Then they presented me with a big gift.

Later the local newspaper ran a short article about the miracle of a dying man returning to life. To this day I don't know what the true diagnosis was.[16]

---

[16] A modified version was first published in *Cortlandt Forum*, "Unusual Case," March 1996.

CHAPTER 17

Am I Losing My Mind?

When a close colleague develops Alzheimer's disease, the author worries if his turn would come any sooner.

It was the Christmas season; time to exchange greetings. So my wife and I decided to visit the local nursing home to meet an old friend, Daniel Jones, MD.

Dan was one of the first surgeons in this charming old southern town of Brooksville. He came from the local medical school, USF School of Medicine, where he taught and practiced surgery for a number of years. Not many American surgeons had wanted to settle down in this "cow country" at that time. But he voluntarily decided to leave his urban practice and come to this sleepy town. When I arrived here in 1981, he had already been in practice for fourteen years. During this period Dan's reputation had gone up, and he was always one of the most sought-after surgeons. Even in his mid-seventies, he was a highly respected surgeon, ever so gentle, and always calm in the operating room. His surgery was clean, the wounds healed well, leaving scars almost invisible, and there were hardly any complications. And he had good rapport with the nurses as well, the epitome of a good surgeon.

When I first set up my cardiology practice, Dan went out of the way to help me. Apart from the usual encouragement and case referrals, he also acted as my preceptor for pacemaker surgeries. No physician on the regular staff, including the three surgeons on the roster, had done a pacemaker implant in our hospital till that time; they were referred to the neighboring hospital. So my request as a medical cardiologist for special privileges to do pacemaker surgery—the entire procedure including the surgical part and implanting the lead all by myself—was not immediately greeted with enthusiasm, but the hospital finally relented with one condition. I should have a preceptor for my first twenty-five implants.

Of course my obvious choice for a preceptor was none other than Dan who gladly accepted the job, knowing there would be no remuneration. I even told him that he could bill for the whole procedure since he was in the OR doing every case with me. And it turned out to be a wonderful and everlasting friendship. I had inconvenienced him many a time, calling for assistance for my surgical procedures, and he always obliged. I developed an abiding affection for this generous gentleman.

Dan was quite a humorist as well. Once, his wife, Sue Ann, had invited us and a few friends for a party. Somebody asked him about his family, and he said: "My three sons are doctors and my brother, Arthur, is a urologist right here in town. My father, of course, was a family physician."

"That is great," I said in admiration. "Three generations of doctors!"

"Oh, it must be some form of hereditary disorder," he said with a chuckle.

One day Dan called it quits and hung up his gloves. He was giving up his slot in the operating room. I bet the other surgeons were happy; one less to compete with. When I ran into him at the local country club a few days later, he was bubbly and cheerful after his golf game. "Hey, my game has improved," he said with a knowing smile on his face. He remarked how he wished that he had retired earlier. He didn't miss the action anymore. He had become a strong voice against the modern trends in the health care industry.

"I am out of bounds for lawyers now," he said with a big grin on his face. "I won't be late in the office anymore."

I reluctantly admitted that there were many who wanted to follow his footsteps. How long can you cope with the doctor-bashing and the new conundrums popping up almost every day in medical practice?

Everything seemed to be cruising well for a while till Mary Ann mentioned that Dan's memory was failing.

"Join the crowd, Mary Ann." I tried to console her. "Sometimes I can't remember some of my own affairs."

"No, no, this is more than that," she said solemnly. Her eyes were getting moist.

Apparently Dan had a full neurological workup and all. The diagnosis became painfully obvious. It was difficult for me to imagine, as brilliant a surgeon as he was, he couldn't remember his name. This man who taught surgery to so many young students, couldn't recognize a scalpel now!

So it was with a heavy heart that I walked into the nursing home. Christmas decorations were all in place and there was a church choir singing carols. The main lounge was glowing with illuminations and decorations. I could see yuletide had arrived. People were warm and friendly.

"Hey, this isn't a bad place to spend your last few days," I said to my wife, secretly hoping I could bypass this journey. I looked for Dan in the assembly there. He was nowhere to be seen. Apparently he was in the west wing. "So what is special about this wing? Surely this must be the VIP wing?" I asked my wife.

I could see the patients were virtually prisoners here. The entry was always locked, mainly for their own protection. Nobody could wander out. We pressed the entry button, and the automatic door opened.

It was a chaotic scene. There were a lot of elderly people in all kinds of activity. Some bolted right to the opening door trying to get out. Others were pacing up and down the corridor babbling away incessantly. I ran into one of my old patients, Rita, who stared at me for a brief moment and then walked away. Suddenly I realized this was their Alzheimer's wing! We went straight to Dan's room and knocked on the door. He was not there. Then we spotted him sitting in a chair, slightly hunchbacked, deeply immersed in thought. He still looked much the same; in fact, more serene than before. He almost looked like an old monk observing his vow of silence.

"Greetings, Dan," I tried to start a conversation, but it was to no avail. No recognition here. Just a curious stare. The flesh looked quite intact but the soul was nowhere in sight. "And how are you today?" I pressed on. "OK." was the short reply.

We gave him a box of Godiva chocolates, which he accepted graciously. I didn't think he knew what to do with them! I felt embarrassed that he didn't recognize me, after so many years of camaraderie. Then he took my wife's hands and started stroking them ever so gently...perhaps an expression of his subconscious love to another human being? He started mumbling something; it was a soliloquy beyond my comprehension. Later Mary Ann dropped in for her routine visit.

"Your wife is here to see you," the nurse announced.

"Which one?" asked Dan without batting an eyelash.

I broke into laughter and soon everybody joined. The tragedy of his mental state contrasted well with the comedy of his words. For a moment I thought this was his humorous self; after all Dan had been married three times and all his wives were still living. I could understand his difficulty. But his blank face proved my assumption wrong.

Suddenly he stood upright and started moving to the corridor. We followed him. He tried to open the closed doors. There were people in some of the rooms. He would gently take their hands, check the pulse, and then move on to the next occupant. Then he quickly returned to his seat, as though nothing happened.

"He still thinks he is doing his daily ward rounds," the nurse said to explain this strange behavior.

I could see that his brain was clinging on to dear shreds of memories. Ideas still fly up from time to time, only to waft away in the next instant. There was a touch of pathos in his face. Part of his brain was still functioning. And yet he was totally lost and helpless. Perfect physical form but a total mental wreck. Once a magician in the surgical suite, he was now reduced to just a shadow of his old self; a physically well-preserved antique but with a big void above. I looked at him again; a stoic but tragic figure. When I called his name, there was no response. Just a glance, a stare. Italians would say *nessun nome*—no name. If his mind was still intact, what would he be thinking now?

Alzheimer's is the most common cause of dementia, the latter defined as "a group of brain disorders that causes progressive loss of intellectual and social skills, severe enough to interfere with day-to-day life." Often the disease strikes people like Dan who are in their upper seventies or beyond, but there is an early onset type that is often hereditary and strikes people in the fifty–sixty age group, sometimes even younger. Fortunately, this variety is rare, affecting only about 5 percent of the population.

The essential pathology is that brain cells degenerate and die, causing a steady decline in memory and mental function. Tangles and plaques appear in neurons from accumulation of a protein called beta-amyloid. It is like a sticky goo that accumulates in the brain and prevents neurons from "talking" to each other. In other words, it causes a disruption in communication within the neurons and hence a block in transmission of stimuli or impulses.

All of us forget a little bit here and there; I do too, which is why I carry cheat sheets and post-it notes to remind myself of the chores for the day. But when it goes beyond that stage with steady deterioration of your acquired skills, it becomes abnormal. In other words, the brain loses its ability for "acquisition, organization, and proper recall" of the experiences in your daily life.

More than 5.5 million Americans suffer from Alzheimer's disease. No doubt, it is a devastating situation, especially for the early onset age group. But it is worse for the caregivers, particularly when the disease progresses and the patient becomes totally helpless. Having treated many patients with advanced Alzheimer's, I empathize with the former because of the complexities involved in the patients' care. And I worry, now that I am getting older, when my turn might come.

"Susheel, where are the car keys?" I asked my wife as we were getting out of the nursing home.

"Don't ask me, you had them last. Where did you place them?" was her cool reply.

"Oh, no…I am not losing my mind, am I?" I said with apprehension.

The fact that I had turned fifty had weighed on my mind for a while. Now that I am over the hump, this could be a harbinger of what is going to happen to me in the future. My introspection got the better of me as I started driving home. Suddenly I seemed to have a broader perspective of life.

I secretly hoped my time wouldn't come any sooner.[17]

[17] February 17, 1988

CHAPTER 18

Doctor-Patient Relationship: Erosion of Trust?

Few things are more difficult in practice than breaking bad news to the relatives of seriously ill patients.

One of the most challenging aspects of medical practice is communication with patients and their relatives, the touchstone for all doctor-patient interactions. Sad to say, this sacred relationship between the doctor and his or her patient has deteriorated considerably over the past few years. There seems to be a constant erosion of this mutual trust, which is why they are asking for second and third opinions. I've had my share of woes as well. Let me tell you about my recent experiences.

Mr. Dugan, a sixty-five-year-old somewhat obese businessman and recently retired, had just moved to my hometown, Brooksville. One morning while he was doing a little gardening, he felt a twinge of chest discomfort and drove himself to the emergency room (ER) of Brooksville Regional Hospital where I practice. By the time he reached the ER his pains had started accelerating, and cold sweats were draining from his forehead. He clearly looked ill.

The first EKG showed definite changes, telltale signs of a massive heart attack, "an extensive anterior wall myocardial infarction" in medical parlance.

"Come quick," the nurse called the ER doctor. "This guy doesn't look well at all."

"Doc, I don't feel good," Dugan said, tossing and turning his head as the doctor started examining him. "Where is the pain, Mr. Du… hey, hey, look at me, Dugan… Nurse, he is coding, come quick, let us start CPR," the doctor was shouting as the patient began rolling his eyes upward and became quickly unresponsive. He needed help and reinforcement.

Two nurses and the respiratory tech arrived promptly. By this time Dugan was in full-blown cardiac arrest and had stopped breathing. CPR was started and a tube was inserted quickly into his trachea and connected to the ventilator. A couple of electric shocks to the anterior chest wall converted the dangerous rhythm, ventricular fibrillation, to a regular sinus rhythm. Once a healthy rhythm was restored with decent heart rate he appeared stable in his current status and was transferred to coronary care unit. However, he remained unconscious

Two of Dugan's sons, executives from Long Island, showed up the next day, deeply upset and furious. They demanded a conference with me right away. They had just one question, "Our father has never been sick a day in his life. He walked into this hospital. Now he is in a coma! We want to know what happened."

I tried to tell them that their father suffered a bad heart attack, went into cardiac arrest, and was successfully resuscitated. I reassured them that he had received excellent care. In fact, the ER crew worked diligently to save his life. Finally, it took the combined public relation skills of the whole staff to pacify the family. I didn't have the heart to tell them that if their father had regular preventive medical checkups and screenings for common cardiac risk factors, perhaps this catastrophe could have been averted. I expected them to be grateful for what we did, but their words implied negligence on the part of the ER staff!

Suddenly my thoughts went back to some thirty years when I was a fellow in cardiovascular diseases at the New Jersey College of Medicine, Newark, New Jersey. One night I was called to see a fifty-six-year-old woman, Vivian, in cardiac arrest. She needed several precordial electric shocks and other ancillary treatments, was on a respirator for three days, in a coma for two more days, and finally survived miraculously. I attended to her earnestly for several days. During her next follow-up visit to the cardiac clinic, Vivian showed me a golden bracelet she was wearing. To my surprise, the name engraved was mine!

And she said: "Thank you for all what you have done for me. You are an angel!" And the grateful family gave me a small gift. Although I generally do not like gifts from patients, since I feel that I am only doing my duty, I couldn't refuse this one because of the genuine feelings of gratitude and appreciation they showed me. So, I accepted the gift with profuse thanks and said, "It was an honor and privilege for me to help you out during this crisis."

Do these two instances tell you something about the changing pattern of doctor-patient relationships? Medicine has certainly progressed through years of spectacular advances that have alleviated human suffering, but what is happening to human relationships? There is a groundswell of dissent among patients these days. Doctor-shopping and doctor-hopping have become all too common. Vivian's story is reflective of a time when the doctor-patient relationship was at its sacred best, when the physician's sincerity and diligence were appropriately reciprocated by the respectful, thankful response of the patient and his or her family.

Over the past decade, innumerable intrusions and incursions have made our practice quite difficult and unpleasant. Gone are the days when a patient will simply accept your advice without questioning its validity. I fully endorse the idea of the patients being educated consumers. However, in many cases, even if you have done the right thing, if they feel uncomfortable in any way with your management style, they may leave you, or even worse, sue you.

Here is another example: Derrick, a thirty-two-year-old man was brought into the ER one evening with severe chest pain that turned out to be from an acute heart attack. Although he had been a pack-a-day smoker since his late teens, I thought he was still young to get a heart attack. On further probing he admitted that he also smoked marijuana and occasionally sniffed cocaine. He was treated promptly with the intravenous clot-buster tPA, and he recovered satisfactorily. Later, on heart catheterization, he didn't appear to have much plaque or any significant blocks, so I surmised that his substance abuse played a major role in bringing on his heart attack.

At discharge Derrick agreed to stay away from cigarettes and drugs, and when he came for a follow-up after one month he appeared to be doing well. His BP was a bit elevated, and he said he had missed out on his medications the last two days. My secretary had already reminded me that he had no insurance and hadn't paid anything toward the large outstanding bill, and she suggested that I talk to him about this.

After the examination I gently reminded Derrick about his bill and indicated that we would reduce the total bill in view of his financial difficulties. I asked him to arrange with the secretary to pay the balance in installments. Suddenly his demeanor changed. He said somewhat angrily, "Hey, man, I don't have any money to pay you. I came to the hospital as an emergency. It is a county hospital, and you know I have been living in this county for the past thirty-two years. I don't owe nothing." He hinted it was my duty to take care of the poor of the county. Before I could say anything further to lighten the situation he stormed out of the office in a huff. I never saw him again.

Later, I got a letter from the public health clinic run by the county to release his records, which I gladly did.

After practicing cardiology for twenty-eight years, I thought I couldn't possibly have any more insights into my own practice, but clearly I was wrong. This case and many others have taught me the evolving mind-set of patients these days. Sometimes, you don't detect any hint of displeasure till you send a bill for your services or get the notice for release of records. The style and semantics of medical practice have completely changed, to say the least.

Few things are more difficult than appeasing the seriously ill patients and their relatives who often do not want to accept your assessment or the bad prognosis that goes with the diagnosis, as in the first case. Transmission of information in an appropriate way has become all the more important to regain respect and faith. Maybe we should look at every situation through the patients' eyes, even though at times they seem very demanding or unreasonable. They do have a pivotal role in all the decision-making processes involving their illness.

In Derrick's case, I didn't quite understand his near outburst when the issue of nonpayment was brought up. By trying to be aggressive with a counterattack, he was practicing the old adage, "Offense is the best form of defense!" He had enough money to buy cigarettes, booze, and drugs but not a dime to pay his doctor who saved his life. I expected something like, "Doc, I will try. I don't have a job, no money you know," but he surprised me with his response.

You live and learn every day, I told myself. As the old saying goes, you win some, you lose some. That is how life is. There will always be Dugans, Vivians, and Derricks in every practice. One must be ready to handle all the situations as they come along.[18]

[18] First published as a modified version in the *Journal of the Florida Medical Association*, October 2005, pg 12-13.

CHAPTER 19

When a Twenty-Three-Year-Old Asks to Die

With nothing more to be done for her, writing a DNR was the humane approach to take. But that is easier said than done, this doctor found.

As I was finishing my office work one July day last year, my secretary told me that I had a consult in the CCU. I went there eager to treat an acute myocardial infarction or complex cardiac arrhythmia. Another opportunity to save a life, I thought. Although a bit tired after a busy day, the prospect of saving a life brightened me.

"What's up, Judy?" I asked the CCU nurse.

"You have a DNR consult in Room 5."

My spirits sagged. DNR orders for elderly patients with Alzheimer's, cancer, or cardiomyopathy are routine enough. But I dislike giving the required second opinion to the physician writing the DNR order. As a cardiologist I'm accustomed to resuscitating patients, and I feel so inadequate when I can't intervene medically to make the patient better.

But this was even worse than I expected. The patient, Angela was only twenty-three. Five days earlier, she had come to the emergency room with pneumonia and impending respiratory failure and was on the respirator. Her history was hardly encouraging. Two years ago she was diagnosed with AIDS. This was her second episode of *pneumocystis* pneumonia, a dangerous, often life-threatening fungal infection, that commonly leads to respiratory failure. And now her doctor has found another microorganism ravaging her lungs.

Dr. David Nielson, the attending, had treated hundreds of AIDS patients. And although he initially thought he could treat Angela's pneumonia, the second infection made it highly improbable that she could be weaned from the ventilator.

My mind snapped back to the moment. Angela's pneumocystis pneumonia was deteriorating rapidly, and worse, another microorganism had been cultured from her body fluids. Her blood oxygen saturation level was dropping and needed more positive pressure ventilation. I could hardly blame Angela for wanting to end this accursed reality. She was lucid at the moment and capable of making a sensible decision. I felt a secret pang as I read of her wish to switch off the ventilator, but inside, I knew that this bedridden existence was no life for a vivacious young woman with ambitions such as hers.

Dr. Nielson, a pulmonologist fresh from Tuft's pulmonary and critical care program, had been attending to her since her arrival. David considered Angela's situation identical to the hundreds of AIDS cases he had seen in Boston and was blunt in explaining that a long-term cure was virtually impossible. However, he was hesitant to accede to the wishes of the juvenile, as he called her, because her condition was potentially remediable with regard to her infection. He was seriously considering switching off the ventilator, but wanted a second opinion from another physician, preferably the chief of medicine. Angela's mother, who had been hovering around her daughter's bed day and night, had been lamenting that she too could not bear to watch her only child in agony as she slowly wasted away to a certain death.

That's where I came in.

After discussing the case with Dr. Nielsen, I decided to go to her room for a physical examination and further talks. She had already been informed that I would be coming and sensed the purpose of this mission. It was indeed a heart-wrenching sight. How a disease called AIDS could transform a young vibrant woman into practically skin and bones. Her eyes met mine; we communicated without words. The pain in her face was obvious; it was more than physical. Perhaps the stigma of contracting such an incurable disease so early in life weighed heavily on her mind.

For a moment I tried to put myself in her position. In fact, only a few months ago I had to undergo a major surgery. Just before I went under anesthesia, I had a sudden surge of emotions. What if I didn't wake up after surgery? I could see some of the events in my life, especially from childhood, parading in front of my eyes. Perhaps Angela was also reminiscing about childhood memories, her relations with people important in her short life, the many unfinished jobs, and unrealized dreams. Does she want to deliberately escape from this world? I wasn't so sure. But then...

How do you withdraw life support from a young woman? I had heard of lawsuits over "pulling the plug," when the family members felt that the afflictions were curable, although the patients themselves wanted to die. This was a thorny situation with legal and ethical overtones. I certainly did not want to provide futile care and prolong Angela's suffering, but I didn't want any legal repercussions either. I had always felt that my mission was to resuscitate patients but the paradigm had shifted here. Frankly I had never been good at handling these terminal care situations.

Suddenly her mother, Vivian, materialized in the room. She must have been waiting for me. Obviously she was crying. Her only daughter was in a see-saw struggle between life and death. I was groping for some words to console her, but none came to my mind readily. Then Vivian started talking.

"Oh, Doc, I don't know what to do. Angela wants to quit. But I am not so sure if she really means it. Isn't there something we can do for her? Is she that bad? No hope at all?"

I didn't immediately answer any of her questions. The whole situation was somewhat overwhelming, and I couldn't make any sense out of it. First I wanted to know what went wrong in Angela's life. Vivian was more than willing to let me in on some of the details. She gave me an old newspaper to read. It contained a detailed story about Angela. Gradually a touching story unfolded.

Angela left home at age fourteen to live with a boyfriend, in spite of disapproval from the family. She didn't complete high school although she was quite intelligent. She jumped from one job to another, changed boyfriends frequently, and drifted further and further away from her family. There was little purpose in her life. But all that changed when she met her new boyfriend, Brian, who would be her future husband. He was a breath of fresh air in her muddled life.

Brian was an energetic young man with a cool head and a balanced mind, just the opposite of Angela. Together they started a restaurant cleaning business in Orlando that flourished. Brian made sure all the bills were paid and some went into savings. They talked about marriage and having children. Angela loved this young man with curly blond hair. Stability and purpose returned to her life, and she was on cloud nine. She reconciled with her family and went back to live with her mom and dad. She had slipped into a comfortable, healthy routine.

One morning Brian showed up at her house and announced that they were driving to the mountains for a mini-vacation. Angela was thrilled and jumped into the car; she even forgot to pack her clothes. Yes, she had worked very hard during the past few months and needed a break. Brian was always so sensible and thoughtful, she thought. It was her dream to spend a few days in the North Carolina mountains. The fresh air would do some good.

Alas, it turned out to be a short ride. In a few seconds, life changed its course completely.

They turned from the side road onto the main highway. Suddenly there was a big bang and a crash. Brian never knew what hit him. It was a four-car collision. Brian's Suzuki Samurai heading north was hit on the front by another car from the opposite lane that crossed the median, totally out of control. A car from behind, unable to stop in time, rammed into the back of the Samurai. There was a fourth car, a Grand Marquis, which also spun out of control, slid into the concrete barrier, launched into the air and headed toward Brian. "Oh, my God," were his last words. Angela passed out momentarily. Neither was wearing a seat belt.

When Angela came to her senses, the entire scene had exploded into a total chaos. "Are you OK?" she asked Brian, but there was no answer. He was lying in a pool of blood, his grossly distorted head practically separate from his body. She was hysterical when the rescue squad and police arrived. She had dragged Brian's head into her lap and was kissing it and mumbling in short bursts: "I didn't even have time to say good-bye to you!"

Poor Angela! In one fleeting moment her life had taken a roundabout. Once the epitome of serenity and stability, her life now was full of tumult and turmoil. She couldn't shake off her guilt feelings. She lost interest in the business. Alcohol occasionally numbed her pains. She again started drifting from one boyfriend to another and had numerous liaisons. Her father was very critical of her lifestyle but couldn't do much about it.

She thought of ending her life a few times but didn't have the courage. She was a small boat aimlessly drifting on the high seas on the verge of a wreck. She had lost the purpose in her life.

Angela had also lost a lot of weight. Everybody thought that this was the aftermath of the accident and the ensuing depression. Once she looked like a model, beautiful and charming. Now her color was gone, and she looked clearly unhealthy. One day she developed a little fever and cough. Vivian took her to a doctor. She had developed pneumonia and was hospitalized. Then came the real shocker; Angela had AIDS! Poor Vivian was totally devastated. But she vowed to take good care of her, and her husband went along with that.

Angela was nursed back to health and her pneumonia cleared. However the luck didn't last long. She had lost her will to live. The ravages of passion were slowly eating her body. The pneumonia attacked her again with more virulence. She progressively became worse, and that was when she showed up in the emergency room.

Now I knew the full meaning of Angela's words when she said, "I want to end it all."

I couldn't agree with her more under these circumstances. I had two options at this point. Since I concurred with the DNR order, I could let them switch off the respirator or I could persuade her to let the disease run its course. I talked with Vivian, then with Dr. Nielson, and again with Vivian. I talked with her priest as well. It was a very difficult and sensitive moment in my life. A young woman's life was in a delicate balance. Once again I tried to look into my soul. Should I prolong her life? Or should all her sufferings come to an end now? No answer was forthcoming. My faith in nature was eroding.

I talked with Vivian, as well as with the priest at length. Dr. Nielson had already made it clear that she could not be salvaged. Angela had had enough and it was time to say good-bye. I couldn't chide her for that. Vivian would go along with that decision. Her only request was to keep Angela alive till her father arrived from New York City the next day.

I promised that I would do my best to keep Angela alive till her father had a chance to see her one last time.[19]

[19] Reprinted with permission from *Medical Economics*: December 11, 1996, 72:23 pg 77-81. *Medical Economics* is a copyrighted publication of Advanstar Communications, Inc. All rights reserved.

CHAPTER 20

These Pains Are Truly from the Heart

A mother finds comfort and solace after taking care of her dying son.

Chest pains are common fare in a cardiologist's office. And many of these patients are referred by family physicians. So when fifty-five-year-old Maureen Palmer walked into the office with escalating chest pains, I was immediately thinking of unstable angina and possibly even an acute heart attack. Since she looked reasonably well without any shortness of breath or sweating, I counted out the latter possibility, but still coronary artery disease was at the top of my list.

A brief history suggested that she suffered from mild hypertension, for which she was receiving appropriate care from her family doctor. "My cholesterol is a bit high, Doctor," she said. "My family doctor suggested that I go on Lipitor but that drug is so costly. I am trying to control it myself with diet. I have started walking more," she added. She looked moderately obese, and I didn't think she was the type who would really indulge in any vigorous physical activity. *The plot thickens*, I thought, what with all those risk factors.

Her husband had died a few weeks before with a heart attack. Before that he was disabled for some time. Her only child, a son named Larry, was living somewhere in New York City. Although gone for almost five years—and never visiting his mother even once—he still kept in touch with her with occasional telephone calls and Christmas greeting cards. Larry was a bit of a drifter, never able to hold down a job, but she loved him anyway. He was reluctant to come back to live with his mother although his mom would have loved it. Still, Maureen was always ready to patronize and support him.

Clinical examination was unremarkable with well-controlled blood pressure, and her electrocardiogram (ECG) turned out to be perfectly normal, not even nonspecific changes (that cliché we all use when we don't know how else to interpret the ECG!) were noted. The rest of the workup, including an echocardiogram and nuclear stress test, did not show any abnormalities either. No evidence of organic heart disease was present. Yes, she did have mild lipid abnormalities but none too severe. I reassured her that she didn't have any heart disease, the stress test especially was quite normal, and there was nothing to worry about. I sent her home with a prescription for a generic statin and a short course of tranquilizers along with instructions on healthy diet and regular exercise.

I thought I would not see her till the next appointment in three months. But she showed up in the office just about two weeks after she left, again complaining of nondescript chest pains. Once again I did a full physical examination, and she was reassured, but she kept coming back with more chest pains. I knew that she was under great stress after the death of her husband, with whom she truly had a love affair for thirty-five years, in her own words. I surmised that perhaps she was still grieving, missing him dearly. On top of that her son was still in New York, constantly looking for a job. Now she lived alone.

My nurse, Rosie, always had this uncanny ability to get into the minds of patients. They always confided in her, and her empathy had earned her more kudos than anybody else in our office. One day I told her: "Rosie, I don't know what is bothering Maureen. Her chest pains are not coming from the heart, for sure. I can't find any cause. She doesn't want to see any counselor. Tranquilizers are not working. What do I do now?"

"Well, Dr. Nathan, Maureen is a little stressed out. Next time when she is around, just ask her about her son; you will see."

"I thought that her son was somewhere in New York, has a job now... right?" Rosy had a nervous smile but didn't answer.

After the day's work was over, in spite of several consults from both hospitals, I decided to call Maureen, wanting to get to the bottom of the situation. It was almost as though she was expecting this call. A "Where have you been all this time?" tone rang in her voice.

It turned out Larry, now about twenty-eight, had recently returned home after five years of living in New York City...with full-blown AIDS! He was just a ghost of his original self. She didn't mind taking care of him one bit...cleaning the bed sheets, sponging his frail body when fever hit him hard, or adjusting the oxygen from the tank. But the thought of losing him, now the only love in her life (even her dog died last year), was much too much for her to bear. Her little Larry had come home to die!

I put Maureen and Larry in touch with our infectious disease specialist, Dr. John Mendoza, and consoled her that she could at least be there for him during this critical period. Fortunately for me, Dr. Mendoza was a very caring young physician who attended Larry well during his last days.

A few weeks after Larry's death, Maureen showed up in the office, with a gentle smile. She appeared somewhat relieved and seemingly had recovered from her chest pains.

"I have no more chest pains, thank God," she admitted.

"I am very happy for you, Maureen. Tell me a little more," I gently prodded her.

Then she told me the whole story about Larry, how he was different from the other kids in the high school, about his illness, and how she had insisted that he come home rather than live in a shabby apartment in the Bronx.

As a parting gift during her last visit to the office, she gave me this compliment: "You are so right, Dr. Nathan. I got the chance to take care of Larry, when he needed me most. I am forever grateful to the Lord."[20]

[20] First published as an abbreviated version in *Cortlandt Forum*, Vol 11 No 12, December 21,1998.

CHAPTER 21

A Tragic Prank

Who would have thought that compressed air could be a lethal weapon, and an innocent prank could snub out a young life?

The year was 1969. I had just returned to India after my postgraduate studies in England. Working in cities like Sheffield, Cambridge, Sunderland, and London, and under the tutelage of a few great professors, I had learned a lot and was quite confident that I could handle any challenges in medicine.

But this one turned out to be quite different.

The first job I got in my home state Kerala was in a large government district hospital in Cochin, as an emergency and casualty physician. I was not fond of emergency medicine but reluctantly took the job since it was close to where my parents lived. During the eight-hour shifts I worked in the ER, there was no dearth of cases. Most of them, though, were run-of-the-mill problems like kids with diarrhea and dehydration, a few cases of nonspecific chest pains and an occasional heart attack, women in labor, and rarely a snake bite or bite from a rabid dog. Oh, yes, there were plenty of motor vehicle accidents, as the number of vehicles on the road had increased steadily without any consideration for expanding the existing roadways. There were a few surgical cases too like appendicitis, gallbladder problems, etc.

One evening, a van roared into the parking lot in front of our ER, and a dozen people in blue factory uniforms spilled out, carrying a young man in great distress. I thought for sure there must have been a major car accident or something, and they were bringing a badly injured victim. They didn't wait for the orderlies to bring in a stretcher or a trolley; instead, a few of them simply carried the patient to the one bed lying vacant in the examining room, skipping all the formalities at the registration counter including the paperwork. This was very urgent, I surmised.

The young man, a factory worker, barely twenty-one years old, looked more like a boy and appeared to be in severe distress. He was writhing in pain. Beads of sweat had welled up along the hairline on his forehead, and his hands were a little clammy and shaking. He was breathing quite fast. There were no external signs of trauma but his belly appeared quite distended.

"This must be a perforated peptic ulcer," I told myself. "So, what happened?" I asked. I was getting a bit nervous myself.

"There was an accident in the factory," a coworker started narrating the tragic story.

"Prepare the OR (operating room). Call the surgeon on call right away and anesthesiologist too." I barked out some orders.

In the meantime, the nurse took his vital signs, and I did a quick physical examination, established an IV line, got several tubes of blood, one especially for grouping and crossmatching, got an emergency chest and abdominal X-ray, and started an infusion of lactated ringer. The nurses and residents were working furiously to get organized, and the operating room was being prepared.

Now the bizarre story unfolded. Anil, just twenty-one years old, had recently joined the local machine tool factory as an apprentice machinist. They worked with pneumatic machines that can emit compressed air jets. His shift was over, and he and his coworkers were in the locker room, getting ready to leave the factory. Anil bent over to pick up something from the floor and one of his colleagues noted a tear in the seam of his trousers between the buttocks. He promptly took the compressed air jet, directed it to the tear, and released the valve. "It was just a prank," he later told me with tears flowing from his eyes. "I intended no harm.

Anil is my friend." Instead of laughing though, the victim screamed with severe abdominal pain and collapsed.

On examination, he was pale, short of breath, quite restless, and thrashing around. He was in agony, breathing quite fast at 40/minute.

His heart was racing at 110 beats/minute. BP had dropped to 100/70.

He didn't have any fever. His abdomen was grossly distended, very tender, and stiff as a board. Bowel sounds, a telltale sign of normal intestinal motility and function were absent, usually an ominous sign suggesting an obstruction or perforation. The usual dullness often felt over the area of liver was absent, suggesting there might be some leak of air. I inserted a finger into his anal canal and rectum but it revealed no laceration or palpable injury. But withdrawal of the finger was followed by profuse discharge of blood-stained fecal-smelling fluid.

By this time the radiology tech came with two films in his hand. I put up the abdominal X-ray on the view box. It was indeed quite revealing, showing extensive pneumoperitoneum (free air in the abdomen). Normally you see only air inside the bowel lumen. Clearly, the patient's colon has been perforated, actually blown up by the powerful jet of compressed air.

Since Anil was in distress, we had to do something quickly. The surgeon would take at least another half hour to arrive. Same with the doctor who had to give anesthesia. The operating room (OR) was not ready yet. *So what should I do now?* was the burning question in my mind. "Do something, please, please," he wailed in a muted tone. Life was ebbing away from him, more from the unbearable pain. The distended belly had to be decompressed somehow.

While the nurse pushed a small dose of morphine intravenously, I cleaned and prepped the anterior abdominal wall and boldly pushed two large bore needles into his distended belly. I couldn't get my hands on a trocar right away. The air, under pressure in the belly, literally whistled out, relieving the distension, and he felt a little better afterward.

The surgeon and anesthesiologist showed up soon, and the patient was quickly taken to the OR. During laparotomy, more air rushed out as the peritoneum was incised and the distended abdomen collapsed. The inside of the abdomen, peritoneal cavity, was grossly contaminated with fecal matter and about 100 cc of blood was sucked out. An irregular perforation of one inch in diameter was present at the lower part of the sigmoid colon that permitted blood and feces along with air to seep out of the colon. There were three additional tears at different sites. The compressed air jet had done its job, tearing apart whatever site it roared through.

The surgeon cleaned the peritoneal cavity, and the sigmoid colon was sutured. After a stormy post-operative course, sadly, the young man bid farewell to all of us. The grieving parents couldn't be consoled.

At the post-mortem examination, the whole abdominal cavity was somewhat disrupted, bloody exudates everywhere, and most of the organs stuck together. The damage was extensive, beyond one's imagination.

Who would have thought that compressed air could be a lethal weapon, and an innocent prank could snub out a young life? But the experts later told me that used in the wrong way at the wrong site in the body, it can be a lethal weapon. Subsequently I did a literature search that told me this type of industrial hazard occurs with gas station attendants, pneumatic drillers, and in any scenario where equipment uses air under pressure. Apparently it is not even necessary for the hose or the jet to be in contact with the body or even the clothing of the victim. The jet of compressed air used in the industry has a pressure of 50–100 lbs. per square inch (your tires in the car have a PSI of only 30–35!), and can generate a lot of force and easily penetrate the vulnerable areas in the body.

I was heartbroken at the sad plight of this young man. A life wasted, all for the sake of a prank. Sometimes life is truly stranger than fiction.[21]

[21] First published in the *Journal of Indian Medical Association*, 1974 62: 7, pg 245-246.

CHAPTER 22

Traumatic Cat-astrophe

Eliciting pertinent historical information is not easy in older patients with their failing memory. So the physician must be especially alert to avoid a misdiagnosis.

Emily was an eighty-three-year-old sprightly woman who lived by herself. She suffered from chronic atrial fibrillation, a rhythm disorder of the heart, common in the elderly, that can lead to such complications as strokes and heart failure. In addition she has been implanted with an artificial aortic valve made from pig's heart called a *Carpentier-Edwards* bioprosthesis, a few years ago. This artificial valve was meant to correct her severe aortic valve narrowing (stenosis) that was not letting enough blood to flow through the tight valve. Both these conditions warranted a blood thinner, and she was put on the commonly used drug, warfarin.

Though Emily initially complained of having too many blood tests, especially the monthly test to monitor her blood thinning time (prothrombin time/INR test, needed to regulate the dosage of warfarin), she finally accepted the inevitable and was doing well. But she never failed to ask me at every visit, "Can't you put me on something else, so I don't have to come here every month for that test, eh?"

Then one day, Emily came to the office complaining of a little pain and swelling in her left groin. "How did this happen, Emily? Did you fall or get hit with something?" I asked.

"I don't remember falling. See, there are no bruises anywhere. Nothing struck me either. Strange thing is, just started coming," she said.

"Any fever, Emily, anything unusual in the stools?" I asked.

I was hoping to get some history that might point me in the right direction. Cancer and infections are commonplace in the elderly population but there was no relevant story forthcoming. Clearly she couldn't remember much about how this developed, but the swelling had been slowly gaining in size over the past few days. Now, it has become a little painful for her to walk. She vehemently denied any history of trauma.

On examination, Emily appeared to be reasonably healthy, without fever or weight loss. The swelling was about the size of an orange, in the left inguinal region. No external signs of trauma, bleeding, or fracture of the hip or thigh was found. Her skin was intact, without any bruises or scratches. There had been no lesions in this area during her office visit three months before. On palpation, the mass was quite hard; in fact, it resembled a rapidly growing tumor in the bone like an osteogenic sarcoma, or metastatic cancer lesion. Her peripheral pulses were all intact and the legs didn't show any vascular problems.

I was quite puzzled as to the etiology of this sudden big lump in the groin. It was quite hard, so the chance of it being a tumor appeared to be high. Emily was sent for an emergency CT scan. And the report came back as follows: "An 8.0 cm mass anterior to the left common femoral artery and left superficial femoral artery is present. It contains a fluid-debris level and does not extend into the pelvis. There is no pelvic lymphadenopathy or masses. Conclusion: hematoma within the left groin."

As soon as I read the report, I telephoned Emily to get a better history. This time I hit pay dirt. Her daughter answered the phone. When I told her the purpose of my call, she said, "Did my mom tell you that she fell in the front yard three weeks ago?"

So there is a history of blunt injury indeed.

With a little encouragement, Emily's memory came back to her. She was able to provide more details:

"About three or four weeks ago, my cat was lying on the lawn. I brought her dinner in a dish, and later, when I tried to take the dish away, she suddenly jumped at me. I lost my footing and fell on a sprinkler head that was sticking up a couple of inches above the ground. I didn't feel anything then and forgot all about it till a few days later when my thigh started hurting. By then, I was due to come see you."

So, that is what happened. The sprinkler head injured the wall of the femoral artery when she had fallen on it and produced a slow leak of blood in the thigh. So, the hematoma was developing slowly over a period of time. The surgeon went to work soon. The large hematoma, filled with several clots and liquid blood, was drained. A small (0.25) laceration of the superficial femoral artery was found to have caused the slow oozing, and it was repaired.

Emily's clinical presentation posed a diagnostic dilemma: a blunt injury that hadn't caused any skin penetration but was severe enough to lacerate the femoral artery, resulting in a slow bleed and a large hematoma eventually diagnosed with the help of a CT scan. Inevitably the corrective surgery was delayed because of slow onset of symptoms, but all is well that ends well.

In the general population, vascular trauma, especially arterial injury, tends to be more common in young adults because they are more prone to acts of violence. However, all age groups can be involved. I tried to look at the literature to get a little more information about these kinds of lesions and found an interesting report. In a large series of traumatic vascular injuries reported from Grady Memorial Hospital in Atlanta, the three most common causes of vascular trauma were lacerations, stab wounds, and injuries from pistol, rifle, or shotgun. Blunt injury was the least common.

An increasing number of vascular injuries occur in the course of diagnostic procedures that necessitate arterial puncture like cardiac catheterization, femoral angiogram, etc. In another large series of acute arterial traumas from Baylor University Health System in Houston, acts of violence accounted for 88 percent of all cases. In a retrospective review of all pediatric patients presenting with non-iatrogenic vascular trauma, the most common mechanism of injury was gunshot wound, followed by stab wound, and the least common was blunt trauma.

External signs, such as skin injury, ecchymosis, or soft-tissue swelling, are often manifest soon after the event. This case was unusual in that there were no such superficial signs that indicated the presence of a deep-seated, serious injury. In older patients who experience blunt trauma, atherosclerotic plaque can further complicate the pattern of arterial injury. Bleeding into the plaque may precipitate thrombus (blood clot) or even dissection (blood penetrating and flowing through the wall of the artery), eventually causing occlusion of that artery, a very dangerous situation.

Vascular injuries to an extremity can result in limb loss, serious life-long functional disability, or even death, if there is misdiagnosis or delay in treatment. Lower extremity trauma with concomitant orthopedic and vascular injury is associated with high degree of limb loss. Despite successful arterial repair, many patients ultimately require amputation, especially if there is a delay in patient presentation. Diagnosis needs to be complete and exact in terms of characterizing the nature and extent of the injury before surgical repair can be carried out appropriately. Arterialocclusive lesions that produce ischemia are generally the focus of initial evaluation, but nonocclusive traumatic lesions resulting in large hematomas may ultimately result in delayed occlusion or the formation of false aneurysms or arteriovenous fistulas.

In older people with failing memory, one needs to be even more alert to the various diagnostic possibilities. Had Emily reported the fall on the day it occurred, we might have detected the hematoma in its early stage. Anticoagulant effects could have been reversed temporarily and even the surgery could have been avoided. Eliciting pertinent historical information is not easy with older patients. One often has to question the relatives who live with them but may not necessarily accompany them to the office. If Emily's daughter had been in the examining room when she showed up, she could have given us the information necessary for the correct diagnosis.

Fortunately for Emily, the hematoma became self-contained, and surgery and a couple of units of blood transfusion cured the problem. But the outcome could have been much worse.[22]

[22] First published in *Cortlandt Forum*, March 1999, 12:3 pg 173–174.

CHAPTER 23

In Remembrance

The treacherous roads claim a lot of lives every year. The untimely death of a beautiful teenager in a traffic accident affected the entire community.

It was early April. When the deputy sheriff knocked on her door, Mary Hawkins gently opened. With a racing heart she asked, "What's the matter?"

"There has been an accident, ma'am, on Highway 50 West," he started in his southern drawl. "Your daughter, Amanda…"

"Is this some kind of April Fool's prank?" Mary asked. She didn't even let him complete his sentence. Her head was reeling, and she almost fainted. She didn't want to know any more.

"I wish it was…" he replied sadly.

"Did you know that Amanda died last evening?" Liza, our friend, called me with panic in her voice. I was shocked. I didn't know that Amanda Hawkins was killed in a grisly car crash on State Road 50. I shook my head in disbelief, because I had seen Amanda on the morning of the accident, driving past our house in her little sporty teal Geo to school, her blond hair put up in a ponytail, a soft smile lighting up her pretty face, and of course, the radio on full blast. I wished the whole thing was just a misunderstanding, but it was not, I knew.

Amanda was a seventeen-year-old senior at Hernando High School who had recently moved with her parents to our neighborhood. They

bought the big, beautiful house at the end of the road. We didn't so-
cialize with them much. But my daughter, two years her junior, had
already become good friends with her. I understood that her father, Tom
Hawkins, was the director of special education in the Hernando County
School District, an important position in this town. Friendly and bubbly,
Amanda always seemed to be driving cheerfully up and down the road in
front of our house. My daughter would often say, "Oh, there's Amanda
again!" Being quite popular, Amanda was a member of an elite clique at
school.

When I left my office on that fateful day around 6:00 p.m. and drove to
the hospital, I was surprised to find that a mile stretch of the high way
was closed and troopers were diverting traffic. I knew something major
had happened, but accidents were not uncommon on these busy roads.
Only later did I realize the magnitude of this one, an incident that would
touch my life deeply.

I contacted my good friend, Mark Jenkins, of the Florida Highway
Patrol, who investigated the scene. He gave me some of the uncomfortable details of this horrific accident.

"Amanda wasn't even at the wheel. Her best friend and classmate,
Kelley, was driving west, in a 1978 MG Midget on SR 50. She swerved
off the road onto the north shoulder. Apparently she tried to return to
the roadway, but I guess she overcompensated and headed straight into
an oncoming sand-hauling ten-wheel 1980 Mack truck!"

He didn't have to tell me the rest of the story. I could imagine. Both
the girls were inseparable to the very end and both departed at the same
time. A purple and gold graduation tassel had been draped over the steer-
ing wheel. On the car's bumper, a sticker declared: ARMY, BE ALL YOU
CAN BE!

Isn't it ironic that life had just ended for these two teenagers? No
drugs or alcohol involved, just a simple human error in judgment. Is this
all the difference between life and death, just one careless moment?

Later, Mark and I were discussing some facts about road accidents in
Florida. He said that for many teenagers, serious accidents are almost im-

minent, because of the way they drive. Some have "one too many" during the parties before they drive home, and the morning newspaper contains the details of yet another alcohol-related crash. Almost every year in this small town, there are at least two or three teenage deaths, victims of horrendous road accidents. Last year, Sherry, one of my friends, had to be flown to Bayfront Hospital's trauma unit after a bad crash, and she stayed in the hospital for three months before getting out on crutches. That touched my life too.

Scores of students at Hernando High struggled with the terrible tidings. "Amanda was, no doubt, *ma meillure amie,*" one of her classmates was heard to comment. Amanda was very active in field hockey and Future Homemakers of America. A good student, she was scheduled to graduate and proceed to college in the fall and become a dentist. Marriage, family, and a new life were all in her plans. But death had cut off all those dreams. The spring break was about to commence, and the kids had some great ideas for their vacation. With tears in their eyes, friends wrote on the lockers in luminescent crayons, "Amanda and Kelley, party on in heaven."

Two days later, I tried to dig into the ugly statistics of road accidents and deaths in Florida for the previous year:

- Among the nearly 500,000 teenage drivers, 317 drivers died in car crashes. And 38 were drinking and driving.
- There were 27 younger than 15 years, and 8 of these accidents were clearly alcohol related.

Teenagers accounted for nearly 5 percent of all crashes.

- Another 17 percent were caused by the 20—24 age group. In our small (Hernando) county alone, there were 28 fatalities.

Now you see the magnitude of the problem.

Just last week, news came from New York that a close friend of mine was killed in a car accident. A drunk driver, a head on collision. It was ironic that this beautiful budding sixteen-year-old, who was attending a prestigious prep school in Manhattan, was coming home from a church service.

Amanda's wake at Brewer's Funeral Home was well attended. My wife and I were there to pay our last respects to a lovely young woman.

This was, understandably, a closed casket ceremony. Later, during the service at St. Anthony's church, nobody could control the emotions...a very large crowd of mostly crying children. They had come to say good-bye to their two best friends. Kneeling in front of the pew, I also said a prayer for her.

After the services, I slowly walked up to Mrs. Hawkins; it was my turn to console her in this most difficult moment of her life. What do you say to a grieving mother after she has lost her precious child? My tongue got all tied up and my brain went numb. All I could do was to gently hug her, briefly telling her how much we loved Amanda, and how I could relate to her pain. There was a look in her eyes that seemed to say, *You wouldn't know what I am going through unless you had been there!*

There is nothing tougher for a parent than losing a child. So full of promise one day and suddenly a collapse of all the dreams. Last year, we mourned young Terry's sad departure in a similar traffic accident. Who is next? How do we prevent this? Can I stand aside and watch as innocent kids fall victims to their own driving? Is teenage driving a lethal habit? Or could it be that a motor vehicle in the hands of a teen becomes a deadly weapon? What do you tell your children when they ask for "wheels" for their sixteenth birthday? Can you trust them with the keys? Can you rest easy till they come back at night?

It seems just when the parents and grandparents need the support and strength of their young sons and daughters, they depart, leaving you to a lonely life. Our teenagers are growing up on the roads! There are rules against drunken driving, not wearing seat belts, and so on. Still the roads claim a lot of lives every year. Can we put a restriction on teenage driving or prepare them better to handle the roads?[23]

[23] September 23, 1993

CHAPTER 24

My Fair Lady

"It is really wonderful that you came from a country from the other side of the world to touch my life and to keep me going for so long with your care and expertise. Thank you..."

After five years as a full-time academic cardiologist at Jersey City Medical Center, a large teaching hospital, I decided to set up a cardiac practice in Florida. Moving from New York City to Brooksville, a small farm town in South Central Florida, was a great cultural shock, and initially I found it difficult to adjust. I missed the teaching, research, and contact with residents, especially the morning rounds, when I got to see them all in one room. For a while I even thought of going back to Jersey City Medical Center, where I could easily claim my job back.

But the rewards of practice that included direct interaction with my patients and, of course, the allure of better income along with the sunny weather kept me going. In any case, winter in New York had become all too difficult for my frail frame to tolerate. So I had no choice except to go south even if the academic atmosphere that I enjoyed so much would be missing. I settled down slowly and accepted the new life.

Then one day Christine McLaughlin walked into my life.

A good physician is not supposed to get emotionally attached to his patients. But Christine became an indelible part of my memory. This sprightly seventy-eight-year-old woman was one of my first patients. She suffered from congestive cardiac failure and had a permanent pacemaker in which she had absolute faith. Mrs. McLaughlin was very sweet, sensitive, and charming, an epitome of gentleness, ever so grateful to her doctor for prolonging and improving the quality of her life. She never complained about the long waiting at the office or the repeated hospitalizations. Her only worry was about George, her loyal, devoted husband of fifty-five years. George, in turn, amply reciprocated her love and affection and often referred to her fondly as "My Fair Lady."

When admitted to CCU once with an exacerbation of heart failure, Christine marveled at the man-made wonders—the cardiac monitors, respirators, infusion pumps, and of course the hardworking nurses and doctors. Even when short of breath from pulmonary edema, her face had a rare grace, serenity, and glow. She rallied and got better, and for a while she appeared to be cruising well.

One day she nearly fainted while tending to her garden. She was promptly brought to the office and evaluated. Interrogation of the pacemaker revealed that it was not capturing well, a sign of impending pacemaker failure. Clearly she needed a replacement, so she was admitted to the hospital for a battery change. With the help of the surgeon, the pacemaker battery was replaced with a brand-new one and her cardiac rhythm was restored. Afterward, she was even more grateful to everybody and everything in life, a rare sentiment in this age. She was thrilled at getting a second chance in life.

On one follow-up visit, Christine gave me a small envelope. Inside was a neatly folded white sheet of paper that contained a poem that she wrote while in CCU, when she was literally dangling between life and death. Her handwriting was still neat and legible, even though she suffered from tremors of fingers and perennial fatigue from her heart failure. As I was about to open the envelope in the examining room, George came from behind and gently touched my back. When I turned around, he told me with a proud and beaming face, "You know, Chris was at one time a nominee for Poet Laureate of Florida!"

I started reading and my eyes became moist.

Life Was Ebbing

My heart remained still
dangerously...until
skillful hands
restored its rhythmic beat.

Now I walk
with measured tread
in coronary cadence and,
count the precious hours

Reaching out to touch my love
I feel in his warm embrace
the merging of his heart with mine,
and our ever present fear."

To this day, I treasure this poem as the most precious gift of all and it hung in my office prominently till the day I retired. Later, she would show me other sentimental poems about her stillborn baby brother, her own newborn, and so on.

It was the autumn of 1984. One day, George brought Christine to my office in a wheelchair.

"You don't feel like walking today, Chris?" I asked.

"I feel weak," she replied, panting, in broken words. "Maybe I belong in the hospital."

From her hospital bed, she admired the live oaks adorned with Spanish moss hanging from all the oak trees outside the window. "That limb is dying, see its withering leaves," she pointed out to me one day with her poetic intuition. She probably visualized her own impending departure from the world she loved so much.

Her condition started worsening. First it was a bad case of pneumonia and then a stroke. More tests, CT scans, EEGs, venipuncture, and so on. Uncomplaining as ever, she still maintained her dignity, stoic calm, and cheerfulness.

Finally it was an open battle with death. Her life and energy were ebbing away every minute right in front of my eyes. One night she slipped into coma. Although anticipated, the reality stunned me. By then, Christine McLaughlin had secured a permanent place in my heart. That day I prayed and prayed for her recovery. The thought that she might not talk or smile or write another line of poetry again struck home hard.

But her time had come. Beside the bouquet of red roses from my garden, which I had brought for her earlier, lay her frail lifeless body. Her last words when lucid were, "It is really wonderful that you came from a country from the other side of the world to touch my life and to keep me going for so long with your care and expertise. Thank you, Doctor Nathan."

"It was indeed a pleasure and honor for me to treat you," I reciprocated.

One of my distinguished professors in the medical school at Trivandrum, India, Dr. K. N. Pai, a great bedside clinician and an outstanding teacher, always used to say: "Patients know their body better than we do. Often they feel it if they are not going to do well, a sense of foreboding."

With her poetic intuition, Christine must have sensed her insidious, relentless slipping into the unknown abysmal nonexistence..."the subsiding of riot of days...the keeping of the last appointment," in her own words.[24]

[24] First published in the Journal of the Florida Medical Association, 1986: 73:19-20.

CHAPTER 25

A Challenge for the Aging Cardiologist

The author faced a true challenge in the ER one day—a morbidly obese woman with very slow heart rate and low blood pressure!

In general, physicians, as they get older, tend to shy away from aggressive and invasive procedures. Maybe one has finally reached a state of equilibrium and gained some degree of equanimity in his or her life and wants to have a little peace and quiet, especially at night. Who wants to deal with blood and gore anymore? Who wants to be called at 3:00 a.m. for a pacemaker insertion or other emergency procedures when you are deep in sleep?

Two of our general surgeons retired at the young age of fifty-three and fifty-four. One opted to become a hospice physician. "You don't have to suffer the wrath of the relatives if there are any complications from my surgery," he said to me one day. The other surgeon decided to pursue his lifelong hobby of playing concert piano. Of course he had received some initial training at Julliard, and he was good at it, so he could still earn an income outside medicine, unlike me.

Many senior surgeons, obstetricians, cardiologists, intensivists, etc., that I know of have become general practitioners or palliative care experts, taking a break from the operating room or cardiac catheterization labs and just offering their cognitive services.

Ever since I turned sixty-five, I have had my share of aches and pains and the end-of-the-day fatigue. Often I have felt the age even though the pundits say, "It is all in the head; you are only as old as you think you are." However, being a full-time cardiologist and intensive care special-ist was becoming increasingly tiresome. Although cardiology was still a labor of love and not something forced upon me, there were days when I would feel it was better to be retired and doing something else. Nearly all friends of my vintage seemed to have retired or were pursuing a less-intensive schedule. Yet, for me, a call from the ER or ICU still gave a surge of adrenaline that I enjoyed very much.

One day, however, I faced a true crisis.

"Doc, I have a patient for you." The ER physician called me in the mid-dle of the night. "Mrs. Hutton, a seventy-two-year-old, with a history of heart failure and renal problems, has a complete heart block. Rate only 20/mt. BP just 80 palp (by palpation). A bit cold and clammy. We will keep her going with the transthoracic pacer for now. Can you get here quickly?"

I had just come back from a three-week vacation to India. The flight alone took over twenty-four hours with a couple of stopovers. It wasn't much of a vacation either this time. I had to do some relief work with tsunami victims and attend two conferences at which I was a speaker. And I was doing all the catch-up work. After a long day at the office and several consults in the hospital, I had come home and just finished a late-night dinner. I was getting ready to hit the bed when the dreaded call came.

"Can you insert a subclavian port for me while waiting? Anyway she needs one with all that hypotension," I gently suggested to the ER doc-tor. A catheter in a big vein for ready access will save me some time and inconvenience as I was gearing for a temporary pacemaker insertion.

"Oh, I am busy, Doc. A couple of trauma cases and a pregnant wom-an in pains here," he said. He clearly didn't want to be bothered.

"OK, I will come soon. Can I do the temporary pacer in the ER, then?"

"Could you please do it in the CCU? We can get her over there quickly; here the ER is very busy today," was his answer.

As I walked into the ER and peeped through the curtain, I knew his reluctance to do anything at this time. To begin with she was a five feet two," three-hundred-pounder! And she had a short neck too, always a barrier for any jugular approach for intravenous line insertions. There was barely any venous access. And right then the lab called with a "panic value" on her blood tests. Serum potassium was critically high at 7.0 mEq/dl, which meant she was probably in renal failure. And that needed to be brought down quickly before she went into a full-blown cardiac arrest. When I tried to figure out where exactly I was going to introduce the Cordis port for inserting a temporary pacer wire I realized my limitations. The right subclavian area had some kind of superficial bruising, and the skin was breaking off. Both her thighs were the size of the trunks of large oak trees I have in my backyard. So it would be difficult to get into a femoral vein also. I had to leave the left subclavian area for a possible permanent pacer. So the only option was to go after the jugular, as difficult as it might be in anybody with short stout neck. And my jet lag hadn't quite resolved either.

In any case, the first thing she needed was a dose of intravenous calcium and sodium bicarbonate and then an infusion of 50 percent dextrose with insulin, to bring down the serum potassium level quickly. I had to use the barely functioning peripheral intravenous line the ER doctor had managed to secure with difficulty. As expected, her potassium came down quickly to 6.0, but the complete heart block and hypotension still didn't budge. Her heart rate didn't improve. Being short of breath, it was difficult for her to lie down flat.

"The BP is dropping, Doc," my nurse said. "It is only 70 palp now."

All right, there was nothing else left for me. I had to get a quick central venous access. "No, there is no surgeon in the house at this hour to do the job," said the nurse after inquiring with the operator.

I put the patient in a Trendelenburg position against her protests, and then struck the jugular vein clean (God must have been watching me closely) in the very first attempt. I threaded the pacer wire quickly and positioned it in the right ventricle. Shortly after pacing was established, the systolic BP quickly came up to 100 mm of Hg, and she started making some urine. Her dyspnea and dizziness abated, and she felt much better. And I got home to catch the much-needed sleep.

Later I reviewed all her medications. Apparently she had been on a combination of many drugs, including one called Aldactone that raises the serum potassium level. Patients who take this drug need frequent monitoring of serum K. On top of that the daughter said: "Oh, I don't know about my mother. She is always complaining of cramps and thinks it's all because of a lack of potassium. She takes sometimes up to nine potassium pills a day."

"She is also quite a bit overweight, don't you think?" I was thinking of the potential problems in doing any procedure on her very obese body.

"My mom has no control over her eating. But it may be because she doesn't walk enough."

Anyway I left it at that. Later one of the daughters came to thank me personally for having saved her mother's life. I sincerely wished the doctor-bashing lawyers and public were paying attention.[25]

[25] February 25, 2005

CHAPTER 26

Serendipity

An astute lab technician's life-saving discovery

Sometimes luck plays a large part in the management of your patients, especially in regard to the diagnosis. Haven't we heard stories of early cancer or heart disease missed, and later they show up with widespread metastasis or a full-blown heart attack. A not uncommon scenario is to discharge a patient who presented with nonspecific chest pain. After the preliminary tests come back negative, the doctor labels the patient as having noncardiac pain, only to see him or her drop dead later from a sudden cardiac arrest. And the most humiliating remark by the patient's relatives is, "Oh, they let him go from the hospital" or "He had only just been to the doctor who gave him a clean bill of health. How come he didn't find anything?" You feel embarrassed and guilty.

However, in the case of Johanna, I was indeed blessed by the goddess of luck, in reaching the correct diagnosis without any delay. It is an interesting story.

Johanna was a seventy-one-year-old slightly obese patient who suffered from mild hypertension and high cholesterol. She was doing OK on medications and her numbers looked good. Her husband, who suffered from cardiomyopathy with mild heart failure, was also my patient. One day she presented to the office with abdominal pain accompanied by cramps, fever, and diarrhea severe enough to warrant hospitalization. She thought that she may have eaten some disagreeable food during the previous night's dinner in a local restaurant.

Clinical examination revealed some fullness and tenderness in the left lower abdominal quadrant, and she looked a bit dehydrated. A chemistry profile on admission indicated a blood urea nitrogen of 32 mg/dl, creatinine 1.6 mg/dl, and random blood sugar 196 mg/dl (normal being < 24, 1.2, and 150, respectively). Initial urinalysis showed a trace of blood and a few RBCs. Urine, blood, and stool cultures to isolate any pathogens were negative, so clearly she didn't have any bacterial infection. And a complete blood count was well within normal limits.

Under a working diagnosis of diverticulitis, Johanna was treated with IV fluids, antibiotics, and painkillers. She had an upper and lower endoscopy that confirmed that she did indeed have extensive diverticular disease of the colon with inflammation around it, called peridiverticulitis. The upper endoscopy revealed a small hiatal hernia with mild inflammation of the stomach lining, called erosive gastritis. Because of Johanna's obesity and abdominal pain, I ordered an abdominal ultrasound thinking she may have gallstones associated with some cholecystitis, although I didn't think strongly that she would have any major abnormality. And the test was scheduled for the next morning.

I was surprised to get a call from the ultrasound technician the following day.

"Hi, Dr. Nathan, I am here with Johanna. The gallbladder looks OK, but I see something interesting below the gallbladder. Don't know what it is. Can I go ahead and do an ultrasound of the right kidney?"

"Yes, of course. But what are you suspecting?" I asked.

"The GB sonogram doesn't show any stones. But my hand kind of slipped down with all this goo around her belly and suddenly I saw the upper pole of the right kidney. Looks like there is a spot there. Need to study it further," she responded.

"OK, go ahead. I will be along, after the office, to discuss it with the radiologist," I told her. Suddenly I remembered that Johanna's urine specimen had shown microscopic hematurea, but I dismissed this as an insignificant finding since the urine cultures came back negative. Anyway this new ultrasound finding piqued my curiosity, and I was eager to see what is going on with her kidney.

Imagine my surprise, when a 2.7 x 2.1 cm solid mass was detected at the upper pole of the right kidney and was further corroborated by a CT scan of the abdomen. Fortunately there was no retroperitoneal enlargement of lymph glands or other signs of metastasis found. A week later, the urologist performed a needle biopsy of the mass and called me after two days with the result: "It is cancer all right, adenocarcinoma. Need to operate soon."

Johanna underwent a right radical nephrectomy, resulting in a total cure. There was no recurrence of the tumor over the next five years while I was following her medically. Then she moved to another area, and I could not follow up.

After Johanna's surgery I reflected on this interesting case. She presented with two serious illnesses, one of which nearly went undetected because of the obvious paucity of clinical manifestations and the dominance of the presenting problem. I shudder to think what might have happened if the alert tech had not detected the lesion in the diseased kidney.

This case reinforced in my mind the role the ancillary staff members play in our professional lives, particularly the technicians and nurses. You never know when they are going to help you save a life. Many times I have depended on the nurses on the floors to help me sort out some of the sticky problems my patients had. Modern-day medicine is a team effort, and every member of the team plays an important role.[26]

---

[26] A modified version was published in *Cortlandt Forum*: An unusual case: November 2004, pg 36.

CHAPTER 27

Sometimes I Feel Like a Pastor!

After many years in practice, I have learned one thing. Listening carefully to patients' stories with a sympathetic ear goes a long way in aiding their recovery.

There are times when my patients simply need an ear to listen to their stories. Often it is about their illness, the stress it generates, lack of family support, and the like. At times they want to vent their gripes about the hospital where they were admitted last time and the not-so-nice treatment they received. And they finish the statement with the remark, "I will never go to that hospital again." All these stories are quite interesting, as they reveal glimpses of their life and all the stresses they face on a daily basis.

Phillip's story

Phillip is a tall, hefty fifty-eight-year-old, who suffered from mitral alular disease and intermittent heart failure. He eventually underwent a valve replacement and has been doing reasonably well since then. He had quite a stressful period during and immediately after surgery but eventually recovered well.

Lisa, his eighteen-year-old daughter, is the apple of his eye. Every visit, he talks affectionately about her. The only problem is that Lisa isn't so caring or loving toward her father and has a wild streak within her.

One day he came to the office as an emergency, looking frazzled and quite tense. He was sweating and fidgety. I could see there was definitely something wrong, and I started worrying about his valve.

"What is it, Phil? Did something happen?" I asked.

"Lisa has done it again. I can't take this anymore." And he started crying unabashedly.

I was a bit taken aback, to see a middle-aged man crying in front of me. My heart went out to him, since I also had a teenage daughter whom I adore. So, I could relate to his feelings.

"My daughter ran away with that wild bunch. She is into drugs. No clue what she's up to," he said between sobs.

"Is this the first time?" I was eager to know.

"No, she does this every so often. Both her mother and I become wrecks, not knowing where she is and what is going to happen to my baby," he added.

I agreed that this was a tough situation for a doting father and very impetuous and self-absorbed behavior on the part of his daughter. Clearly she needs to get off the drugs and stay away from the bad company She will need a lot of psychological counseling. And of course, some detox too. I sat him down and gently patted his back; my nurse came in and gave him a glass of water. He calmed down a little. Then I gave my suggestions to improve the situation.

"First you need to report this to the police. It is urgent, especially since she is into drugs and bad company. Once she comes back, you and your wife need to talk to her lovingly as you do, and make her realize how this is affecting your health, and it is certainly not good for her future. Then get her to a detox or rehab center. She will need strong psychological counseling and your support," I said earnestly.

He appreciated my taking the time to talk to him and left the office in a better state of mind. And I realized it is tough enough when you have a significant cardiac problem that can get worse at any time, especially when subjected to severe stress like this. On top of that if you have to handle such egregious behavior from your children without any consideration for their parents' welfare, life can become miserable.

Sophia's story

Sophia is a middle-aged woman whom I follow regularly for hypertension. Her husband is in his late fifties. Only once have I seen him with Sophia. Often she comes alone. Always cheerful and smiling, she inquires about my wife and children as well as my welfare. So I was surprised to see Sophia a bit gloomy and not her usual self when she came for a follow-up one day.

"I am really sad today, Dr. Nathan. Maybe I need your advice." She started talking even before I got a chance to say anything.

"What is the matter, somebody sick at home? Is your husband OK?" I asked her gently.

"My husband is *the* problem, Dr. Nathan. I don't know what to do," she said plaintively.

"Maybe I can help. Is it a cardiac problem?" I asked, hoping I could offer my services as a cardiologist. I couldn't be certain if it was a marital issue as well.

"It is not what you think. You wouldn't believe it. My husband ran away a week ago. And you want to know with whom?"

Just when I thought there was another woman involved, she dropped the shocker.

"It is another man, a man, Dr. Nathan!" she said with a sarcastic tone. "He is only an eighteen-year-old boy. They went to Philadelphia together.

I wasn't really prepared for this strange twist of events in her life. Marital disharmony, conflicts with the proverbial other woman, difficult divorce proceedings are so common in our society. One hopes those things do not happen after so many years of successful marriage, as in the case of Sophia. So, I was perplexed for a moment, unable to absorb the impact of this new conundrum in her life, and I was at a loss for words to advise her.

"Have you tried to contact him? Did he leave a note or something?" I said.

"Oh, what is the use? He called me yesterday only to say that he is moving out, will come back to pick up the stuff and sort out some matters," she said with resignation.

I said, "Do you both want to go for counseling? Make an attempt to patch up your differences. You don't have to give up that quickly. What do you think?"

"It is not going to work. I know him well by this time. He has made up his mind," she added.

"Well, then, maybe, it is all for the best. If he is bent on leaving you, he will. You need to get on with your life. Try to make the split amicable," I tried to console her.

Finally she accepted my suggestions to do whatever is necessary to have a smooth divorce. "Well, do I have any choice?" she asked me as she was leaving the office.

Terry's story

Terry, a prisoner at the local calaboose, was admitted to our ICU. He looked quite weak and ill, with fever and weight loss. The admitting doctor was worried about infective endocarditis. He was chained to the bed and a deputy was sitting next to him when I came to see him. Obviously he was under protective custody. And his crime, "Oh, he was shooting up drugs in the alley, and we were called in by some neighbor because of the altercation and the noisy quarrels in the area. He was resisting arrest and is now charged with assault on an officer."

When I examined him, Terry appeared to be quite ill and very depressed. He had a pathetic, hopeless look about him.

"I drink a bottle of rum or whiskey, whatever I can get. Sometimes more. And I smoke up to three packs (cigarettes) a day," he said. "Oh, I shoot drugs too, i.e., whenever I can get my hands on some," he added.

The nurse had told me earlier that they had found some drugs on him."

"Why, Terry, why? Are you trying to commit suicide?" I asked with sincerity. "At this rate, you won't last too long."

"Oh, what do I want to live for? I have nothing to look forward to. I just want to live *till I see my brother and sister dead!*"

I almost had a double take. But he meant it. Obviously it was a sour family relationship. "They are older than me, but they never did any good to me. I was always the bad boy in their eyes."

"How about your wife?"

"Oh, I left her long ago, thank God. She wasn't any good either." He didn't expound.

I reviewed his chart in detail. He was clearly septic with intermittent fevers. He looked unshaven and unclean, febrile, and self-neglected. Chest X-ray report showed pneumonia in one lung, and tests for AIDS were still pending.

Clearly, Terry was in bad shape, and I was worried that his wish may come true. So I sat down with him and started counseling. "Terry, the past is past, and we cannot erase it. But at some point in life, you need to start the recovery and rehab process. I agree the road to recovery may not always be smooth or straightforward, but you need to start at some point. This is the best time to do that while you are in the hospital. And we will try to do our best to get you out of this predicament. And our social services will help you to get back on your feet."

There was a gentle smile on his lips. Was he thinking that a new day had dawned in his life, beginning of a new life perhaps, healthier and happier than before? Or was he thinking of the futility of all what we are doing for him? I would never know; after a few days he was transferred back to the jail and was lost for follow-up.

Elaine's story

Elaine is fifty-five and is actually running for the county commissioner's position in our small county. One day, during her regular office visit, she talked about her frustrations in life. And there appeared to be quite a few. She had to cope with her own illnesses like hypertension, diabetes mellitus, and a little obesity. When I gently taunted her about not losing weight after much counseling and dietary instructions, she gave me her standard reply: "Oh, I am trying, I am trying, Doc, but this weight won't budge! And you know, my husband is not well either. I have to spend a lot of time taking care of him. So I have to eat on the run often. And my daughter is having problems too."

Her twenty-four year-old daughter, Doreen, who had a two-year-old child, was getting divorced from her thirty-year-old husband.

"Doreen has been married to Glen for three years, and I have an adorable grandson. She found out Glen is cheating on her. I don't even want to call him my son-in-law. He is actually living with another one! I wish they hadn't gotten married. Now my husband and I need to take care of her. Actually Doreen and the little boy are living with us." There was sadness in her voice.

"Did they go for counseling? What is Glenn's stand? Who will take care of the boy when Doreen has to go to work? It may not be too late to patch up the differences," I said in an attempt to give her some comfort. As an incurable optimist I was trying my best to salvage this broken marriage and the complications about to unfold.

"Oh, it is a hopeless situation…it would be better if they can get it over with and move on with their lives," Elaine said with a deep sigh. Clearly she was under great stress.

"Well, in that case, Doreen can go for counseling, let the lawyers handle the divorce situation. Divorce is commonplace, it is not the end of the world," I tried to reassure her.

"I know you have a lot on your plate now. But we all have to carry our cross sometimes. It is better to reconcile with the situation, do our best, and then move on," I finished my little sermon. "And best of luck with your campaign," I added. She appreciated my words.

Sonali's story

Sonali was a true challenge indeed.

She walked into my office one day and literally slumped on the examination table. "You better see this patient first," my nurse said. "She doesn't look so hot."

Yes, Sonali was a bit short of breath, looked pale, washed out with a puffy face and a wan smile. She looked quite anxious too. Her pulse was fast and the veins in her neck looked abnormally gorged and unhealthy. I knew she was clearly sick, quite sick?

After the introductions, I asked, "What is going on, Sonali?"

"Oh, it is a long story. I will admit it, I am an alcoholic. What can I do, you tell me?

"Oh, my husband, he is a rascal, he never supported us, cheated on me, and I threw him out. He would never work. I had a job, but I lost it after my drinking started. I tried it at first to drown my sorrows, but now it has become a habit."

It looked like it was more than a habit. She looked like she was "preserved" in alcohol. Her sixteen-year-old daughter, Sheena, was already fed up. She looked more mature than her age, perhaps the result of having to take care of an ill mother and shoulder other responsibilities in the house at such a young age.

"The only time Mother goes out is for a beer. Then she sits and drinks or just sits and sulks. There is no money, and we don't have many friends to ask for help," said Sheena.

"What about your grandparents? Can't they pitch in?"

"Oh, they are in Puerto Rico and can't help much," she said sadly.

I suspected that Sonali was suffering from congestive heart failure and hence admitted her to the hospital and started her on a full decongestive therapy. It turned out that she had severe cardiac damage from chronic alcoholism and all we could ask for at this time was to stabilize the condition; hopefully she would continue to improve once she quit drinking. Within a few days she felt better and her breathing problems abated. With home health care and intervention from social services, she stabilized. I gave my usual sermon about throwing away one's precious life at such a young age, especially since she had a disease eminently treatable unlike metastatic cancer (that is my usual spiel!). And of course she needed to care for a young daughter too.

With proper rehab, home health services, and a little extra motivation she eventually got rid of her alcohol problem. The next time she came in she appeared better. She promised that she would do her best to stay healthy, and I counseled her about staying dry and taking up some of the responsibilities of a mother. I also told her that she should be proud of her teenage daughter. Once she has remained dry for at least six months, I promised to send her to our cardiac transplant program at Tampa General Hospital in Tampa for evaluation and eligibility. I had to counsel the daughter too, who promised to keep an eye on her mom.

After many years in practice, I have learned one thing. Listening carefully to patients' stories with a sympathetic ear goes a long way in aiding their recovery.[27]

[27] Written at different times: 2000—2009

CHAPTER 28

Looking for
Alka-Seltzer

One patient was lucky that he ran out of Alka-Seltzer and was forced to come to the hospital, because this indigestion turned to be quite different.

Larry was a fifty-two-year-old, successful executive at a local company who also had a roving eye. So his wife kicked him out of his house, and he was temporarily living with his girlfriend, a young nurse, in a motel close to our hospital. He often would ride around the area on his bicycle for exercise and hadn't experienced any problems like chest pains or shortness of breath. A little on the obese side he hadn't suffered from high blood pressure or diabetes.

For some time though, he had had bouts of indigestion that were easily relieved with Alka-Seltzer. So he always kept a supply in his room and carried a few tablets with him on his journeys. Not one for having tests, he was very confident of his good health and rarely saw his family physician.

One Friday night, while watching TV, he fell asleep but woke up about 10:00 p.m. with a little heartburn and indigestion. He reached for his pills and found he was fresh out of Alka-Seltzer. He opened a can of light beer and took a couple of gulps and decided it didn't taste good, so he tossed the can into a trash bin. His girlfriend had taken his car away to the hospital and wouldn't be back till the next morning. These days she was on night duty.

For a moment his thoughts were, "What do I do now, go to Publix and get some pills or go to Brooksville Regional Hospital?" The hospital was only a mile away and would be an easy ride on his bike, so he decided to take the short trip to the hospital emergency room on his bike. "It shouldn't take much time, just get a couple of antacid pills and come home," he told himself And he took an aspirin before he started on his bike, hoping the discomfort would ease a little.

The ER as usual was quite busy and so he cautiously approached the front desk and asked the clerk: "Can I get a couple of pills for my heartburn? I ran out of my Alka-Seltzer," he said.

"Sir, you have to register first, need your name and insurance, etc.," the clerk advised him.

"Is that really necessary? You know, I get this all the time. Don't want to trouble you much," Larry said meekly.

The clerk called the nurse to handle the situation. She was in charge of triage, and she would evaluate the patients first and decide which patients needed to be seen pronto, as suggested by their symptoms.

The nurse promptly came out to the counter and asked him politely, "What seems to be bothering you, sir?"

"All I need is a couple of Alka-Seltzer, just have a little indigestion."

"We can't just give you Alka-Seltzer. Need to check you out first," she said earnestly.

"Oh, my...do I really have to have a checkup? You know, I get this every now and then." Larry tried to impress on her that this wasn't all that serious as they seemed to think.

"No matter, hospital policy" she said firmly. "Besides, we can't be certain if this is due to something more serious." The nurse was insistent.

"Aka-Seltzer relieves my heartburn all the time, and I really don't want to go through all that," he appealed once more.

She, however, persisted with her request and finally persuaded him to come inside and get checked. Although he was a little skeptical, Larry went along with that.

"No point in going back, especially since my woman is not in the room," he said to himself.

His vitals were normal. The nurse then proceeded to do an EKG and shouted some orders to one of her colleagues about a few quick blood tests. "Just tell the doc that I have a new patient here, and I am doing the EKG now," she said.

A big surprise was awaiting Larry. A twelve-lead electrocardiogram showed an acute, extensive, anterior wall myocardial infarction (MI).

"Doc, come here quick. This gentleman is having an acute MI. The EKG shows some pretty big changes. Looks like the STs are going up!" She couldn't contain her excitement and anxiety.

The doctor sprang into action and so did the entire ER crew. Larry was immediately examined, and the doctor confirmed that Larry indeed was having an acute anterior wall myocardial infarction. I was the on-call cardiologist, and he apprised me of the situation. I told him to proceed with the emergency treatment tPA, a clot-buster, intravenously followed by Heparin, a standard combo for the treatment of acute MI, and all the other ancillary treatment for the condition. Primary angioplasty (opening up the offending artery by urgent cardiac catheterization) was not available in those days in our hospital. He was then moved to the CCU and closely observed and monitored. I saw Larry in the ER itself and later in the CCU. And then I left a message with the CCU staff that I wanted to talk to the family in the morning before I went home.

The following morning, Larry appeared to be doing well. "Where is the wife? I wanted to talk to her," I said to the nurse.

"Oh, Dr. Nathan, both his wife and girlfriend showed up. You missed all the fun. Those two ladies were going at each other's throats, and I threw them both out. They must be in the waiting room. They both want to see you."

I called both of them separately and apprised them of the situation.

A few days later, we did a cardiac catheterization and angioplasty of the left anterior descending artery. Needless to say his "indigestion" was cured.

In spite of all the advances we have made, nearly half a million people die suddenly each year from heart attacks in this country. A good majority of these lives can be saved if appropriate treatment can be given in time.

It was pure chance that Larry ran out of Alka-Seltzer at a crucial moment and decided to go to the ER to get more antacid. And it was his good fortune that a vigilant mind steered him in the right direction once he was in the hospital waiting room. Taking the aspirin before he hopped on his bike was the right thing to do if he was developing a possible heart attack, although he was not aware of this recommendation put forward by AHA. Missing an acute MI can prove to be deadly.

Larry survived the crisis and went on to live well afterward. I don't know if the wife and girlfriend reconciled after their showdown in the hospital.[28]

[28] A modified version was first published in *Cortlandt Forum*, June 1998, pg 43.

CHAPTER 29

The Last Stretch

A long awaited opportunity to receive a life saving heart transplant finally arrived. However the patient's reluctance to quit smoking turned out to be a major road block in achieving the goal.

December 2008

The first time I saw Peter was in the emergency room of Brooksville Regional Hospital. He was admitted with severe chest pain one evening and the ER doctor wanted a cardiac consult right away since there were some changes in the electrocardiogram (EKG)—signs of a possible heart attack, he thought. Although I was getting ready to go home, this consult took priority, so I hurried to see him. As I stepped into the ER, the nurse came running and said, "This guy is a regular here. He comes in with the same problem. You know he fired his previous cardiologist. Now he wants you, lucky guy!" She winked at me and went back to her station. Was there a hint of warning in her voice? If I can't go along with what he wants, he might fire me too.

I gently pulled the drapes around the bed and introduced myself. Although Peter appeared to be short of breath and on oxygen, he acknowledged my presence with a feeble "Hi." He was almost cold and clammy, and very anxious. The ER doctor came with his EKG and said, "Look, the second EKG shows a lot of changes; looks like he is having acute anterior wall myocardial infarction (a heart attack in the front wall of the heart, quite serious)." He was obviously right.

"Why didn't you call the interventional cardiologist right away?" I asked the doctor. "You could have saved some time." I was a noninvasive cardiologist. Sometimes I jokingly tell my colleagues that I am an "evasive" cardiologist who prefers not being consulted for very difficult problems.

"You were on call, plus the primary mentioned your name," was his answer.

In any case, Peter was rushed to the cath lab. My colleague, Dr. Thomas, was still in the house. The cath was completed quickly, and he called me from the lab.

"Oh, your man has severe disease of his native vessels. All the three (coronary) grafts are gone. No definite lesions that we can dilate. It is just terrible disease everywhere. And oh, his LV (left side of the heart) is not so hot either. I get an EF (pumping fraction of the heart) of just about 15 percent. That is pretty bad. You know he has an ICD (implantable cardioverter defibrillator) already, right?"

After transferring the patient to the CCU and starting him on the right therapy, I studied his old charts. He had several hospital admissions for one thing or another, mostly for chest pain and heart failure but also for chronic respiratory problems. His cardiac problems dated back in his late forties, and he'd had a triple vessel bypass surgery at fifty-two. In spite of strong advice from all the doctors, he continued to smoke and drink. No wonder that his heart muscle became weak, and he started slipping into heart failure. After a few episodes and a close brush with death from ventricular tachycardia, a life-threatening heart rhythm disorder, he was implanted with an ICD.

The pulmonary physician, Dr. Shah, was already at his wit's end because Peter wouldn't quit smoking despite severe emphysema. His lungs began to fail. He wasn't a compliant patient in other ways. When he ran out of medications, he wouldn't call for a refill. His wife wasn't always very cooperative nor was she very supportive of his needs. I wasn't certain if I wanted to follow him after discharge since my experience told me that such noncompliant, restless patients become disenchanted with one doctor and move on to the next one. But at the request of Drs. Meehan and Shah, I agreed to follow him in the office. But I didn't harbor any illusions that I was going to make him much better, nor would he listen to my instructions.

January 2009

During the first office follow-up visit, I sat down with Peter and his wife, Gloria, and explained the current situation. Gloria was also a smoker.

"Why haven't you quit smoking yet? You know your heart is getting weaker every day from all the poisons you inhale from the cigarettes?" I asked.

"Believe me, I'm trying. But you don't know how difficult it is to get off of it. Did you ever smoke?"

I smiled. I knew this guy was not going to quit anytime soon. Then he surprised me. "OK, give me that latest one, what is it called, Chantix? I hear it's pretty good."

"I will give you a script if you want; it is a bit costly. But both of you have to quit together, if you really want to quit for good," I warned. Gloria turned her face the other way. I knew what that meant. "Oh, one more thing, if your heart muscle function doesn't improve much, you may need a new heart," I added. Peter brushed it off as a joke, and I didn't want to push the issue further.

March 2009

With an optimal regime of medical therapy, constant home care, quitting smoking, and significant modification in his diet, Peter seemed to be making some improvement. But his cardiac function continued its downward slide. So one day I broached the issue of cardiac transplantation again with his wife intently listening. I didn't see any alternative to tackle his universe of problems.

"You know, Peter, your heart failure is getting worse. The only option we have is to consider cardiac transplantation. Do you know what that is?"

"What does that mean?" He looked puzzled. But Gloria caught on to the idea quickly.

"Well, I am talking about a cadaveric heart transplant. Yes, getting a new heart from somebody who died recently. It used to be an exotic treatment, but now it is done routinely. Yet I must warn you it is not easy to get one. Only about two thousand heart transplants are done yearly in the US. Several thousand are waiting. You have to be ready and willing to go through the surgery at a moment's notice."

Both of them appeared to be very interested, so I decided to make a call to Dr. Jason McDaniel, the chief of cardiac transplant surgery at the university hospital in Tampa. We knew each other well and he agreed to see him for an evaluation.

For Peter, the next few weeks were punctuated with more tests, frequent trips to Tampa, a drive of fifty miles from his home—which his wife didn't enjoy—psychiatric evaluation, and finally review by the entire transplant team. Since suitable hearts are difficult to come by and criteria for inclusion are stringent, most people get rejected.

Then one day, the much-anticipated call from Dr. McDaniel came. I took the phone with a little apprehension.

"Hi, Dr. Nathan! I have good news. The transplant advisory group at our university hospital agreed to put him on the list. One stipulation, though: he can't smoke or drink anymore. We have informed him quite strongly."

Peter was given the usual instructions and given a special beeper that would alert him whenever a new heart became available. Then he would have to be rushed to the operating room. I also told him, "From now onward, I will act as your local cardiologist for emergencies only, so you keep in touch with Dr. McDanielWeston. Whenever there is a major problem, he needs to know right away. You will have to make many trips to Tampa."

May 2009

A few weeks later, he was back in the ER. This time it was his ICD that was firing intermittently giving him small shocks in the chest. Obviously, he was having recurrent episodes of ventricular arrhythmias that got shocked by the ICD. The electronics specialist from Boston Scientific analyzed the device and confirmed that he did have an episode of ventricular fibrillation (a fatal arrhythmia if not converted by electric shock) that was corrected with one shock of thirty-one joules strength, delivered automatically by the implanted defibrillator. He received one more under similar circumstances a few hours later. "Oh, the device is working well, it is doing its job," he said after interrogating the ICD. Peter got a slow infusion of potassium intravenously since the level of this electrolyte in the blood was quite low. He became stable, but needed intravenous Primacor therapy to support his failing heart. Finally, he was sent home, although I knew his destiny was sealed if he didn't get a heart quickly. I felt this was the pinnacle of my efforts.

Soon I was on the phone with Dr. McDaniel, apprising him of Peter's current status and how urgent the situation was. "I don't know how long he can last this way," I told him with great concern.

"Yes, looks like he is getting closer to the end. Let me see if I can bump him up on the computer," he said wistfully. "You know how hard it is to get a matching heart in good shape," he reminded me.

Two weeks passed with no news from Peter or any call from the ER. I was beginning to relax, thinking that perhaps Peter was stable, at least for now. The home health care sent me periodic reports about his vital signs and his general progress, detailing his breathing patterns, status of congestion in the lungs, etc. And the home IV infusions were going well. However, in one of the reports the nurse mentioned she couldn't be sure if he had started smoking again. So I called her to verify.

"You know, the other day when I walked into the house, I could have sworn there was the smell of cigarettes in the air. But both of them promptly denied. Dr. Nathan, I don't trust either of them. Gloria was almost offended when I hinted about it. You ask him yourself next time," she said.

June 2009

A week later, the couple showed up in the office for the scheduled follow-up. It wasn't quite a happy scene. Peter was panting, unable to catch his breath and his oxygen saturation had dropped considerably. It was already low in spite of home O2 therapy. Gloria was restless and upset. Her question was, "How long can he last like this? They better get that heart for him."

I tried to explain. "You see, Gloria, it is not that easy. The transplant team is doing all they can. His name has moved up in the computer, thanks to Dr. McDaniel. But it is anybody's guess when he will get a suitable match."

She grumblingly accepted my words. Then I popped the question, "Has he started smoking again?"

"Why do you ask?" she immediately retorted, obviously looking irked.

"His O2 sat has dropped and the home health nurse was concerned. His heart failure is getting worse," I said.

Gloria looked down, not wanting to make any comment.

"I am not sure if they would keep him in the program, if he doesn't quit. What about his drinking status?" I asked.

Gloria hesitated for a moment. Then, uncharacteristically, she opened up, tears welling in her eyes.

"There is no point in hiding the truth from you, I guess. He is doing all those things again! He smokes at least a pack a day, maybe more. And polishes off a few beers too every day," she confided.

"That explains the worsening of his condition. Have you had any calls from the university hospital or Dr. McDaniel lately?" I asked.

"Well, yes," she started reluctantly. "Peter was in Dr. McDaniel's office last week. They did a bunch of tests, some for his lungs too. We were told he is going downhill fast. Only 10 percent of his heart is working now!" Then she clammed up, looking glum.

"So, did they say he was moved up in the computer?" I was eager to know.

She hesitated and then dropped the bomb, "They took him off the list!"

That landed like a fist in my face. We were silent together for a few minutes. I tried to digest the idea.

"Took him off the list? Did they give you a reason?" I asked finally. I had given so much hope to this couple, they were banking on getting a new heart. And Peter was only fifty-nine, too young to die, I told myself. His life was being held together with a patchwork of drugs and devices.

"Well, Peter isn't as innocent as you think, Ravi," Jason said when I called him as soon as the patient left my office. "To begin with, he missed two appointments here. He is under close surveillance when he is on the waiting list and while getting Primacor infusion. On top of that he started smoking and drinking. I am not sure if he is even taking his meds regularly. So we had to make a decision."

I was a bit overwhelmed at this sudden turn of events. "This is so tragic," I said. I felt for my patient, although his behavior lately had not been very honorable.

"You know we can't waste a heart if the patient is not cooperative and doesn't understand the logistics involved in procuring it, the surgery, and what comes afterward."

"I understand," I said, my voice cracking.

"OK, I can still put him back on the list, but only after he totally quits smoking and drinking. And yes, he has to take his meds regularly and must keep his appointment in the office diligently. "No show in a transplant clinic is a no-no," he added.

I called Gloria right away to come back for a discussion.

"You mean he'll get another chance?" Gloria's eyes widened when I told her what Jason had told me.

"Well, if he can quit his booze and smoke, maybe," I said.

"Leave it to me, I am going to hide all his cigarettes and bottles," she said emphatically.

"That will be a good start. But first you have to quit too; otherwise, he will want to light one up whenever you do," I warned.

"I am going to give it a try. He is all I have," she said.

With help from the home health nurse and encouragement from his wife, Peter was weaned off the cigarettes and booze one more time. Then he had to be admitted to the hospital for worsening heart failure. He spent his time in the ICU, a place he had become quite used to. He knew all the nurses on a first-name basis. When he was stable again, I called Jason and asked him to consider putting Peter back on the list.

"Let me bring this up in the next committee meeting. The committee makes the final decision. But I'll give my nod. Ravi, please understand we are going by your word."

July 2009

I did not hear from Peter after his discharge, for two weeks. He missed his one-week follow-up appointment, and I was too busy to call him back. Being on call for one whole week for our ER was not an easy matter. Acute heart attacks, life-threatening cardiac arrhythmias, rapidly decompensating hearts, cardiac arrests…there was no dearth of emergencies. Some days I really felt like throwing my beeper away.

While rounding later that week, I got a call from the ER. "Your patient is here, you know whom I am talking about …. Peter Slades."

"How bad is his heart failure? Is he in severe pulmonary edema?" I anxiously asked.

"Oh, he's here with hemoptysis" (coughing up blood). "His INR (blood thinning time, a marker to evaluate the effectiveness of warfarin therapy) is way above the normal range."

I broke my ward rounds and rushed to the ER. Indeed, Peter was coughing up blood in his sputum from a combination of his pulmonary congestion and excessive effect from warfarin therapy. After a large dose of Lasix (a diuretic) along with adequate respiratory therapy, he felt better. Then I asked him, "How come your INR is out of whack? Did you take anything other than what I prescribed? Like antibiotics or pain medications? I was thinking of other medicines that might prolong the effects of warfarin.

A quick call to my office revealed the dose of warfarin prescribed. Peter insisted, "No medicines other than what you had given me." But my secretary said there was a note from the home health nurse that suggested that the patient or the wife didn't seem to know much about the drugs or the dosage and may not be taking them properly. Later, when she went by to check the INR, Peter wasn't home. "He has gone urgently to see one of his relatives and won't be back for a few hours," she was told. She advised him in vain to come to the office to check his INR.

The blood results showed that his INR was indeed twice the therapeutic level, suggesting blood was thinner than normal, which explained at least partially why he was having bloody sputum. This occurs from a minor rupture of the alveoli or bronchial cells in the lung, on coughing. Although he didn't have the dreaded pulmonary embolism and pneumonia, his lungs were congested. Finally, with a few days of ICU treatment and drug adjustments, he went home again. I informed Jason about this setback, and he said, "Well, I don't know, Ravi. If he or his wife cannot pay attention to his medications now, how is he going to handle the drug regime after transplant? Anyway, let him come back and see me as soon as possible, maybe within a week."

During the next several weeks, Peter steadily went down. He also appeared to be disenchanted about his future prospects. Gloria was also unusually passive. At the time of discharge, I had impressed on him what needed to be done, keeping a close check on all medications taken, frequent lab tests, the importance of keeping appointments both with my office and with the transplant cardiologist. I also arranged home health care services to monitor his vitals, medication intake, and lab tests. I thought both of them understood the gravity of the situation.

Two weeks passed. Peter missed his appointment in the office again. When my secretary called his home, there was no answer, so she asked the home health nurse to check on him. We were worried that he had collapsed and was lying around somewhere. The next day the nurse called me.

"Peter is at home, all right. But guess what, he is smoking again, and I just wondered if he smelled of alcohol too. I really don't know what is going on with that family." So I asked Gloria to bring Peter to the office the next day. She reluctantly agreed.

This follow-up visit didn't go very smoothly.

"What is going on, Peter? First you missed the appointment here and then in Tampa. Now you have started smoking and drinking. Do you remember what I told you earlier?" I asked.

Peter had a distant look in his face. Gloria looked disinterested.

"I don't know what is happening," he said. "You tell me. One day I am OK, but the next day I can't catch my breath. And I take all these drugs that cost me an arm and a leg; what for?"

"Listen, Peter, I told you so many times. Your heart has no reserve. You can't smoke and drink anymore. If you want, I can prescribe you the nicotine patches or gums."

"I can't afford those costly goddamn patches! No way!" he said.

"Are cigarettes any less costly? Anyway, you had quit once, you can do it again," I said. "You were sober, they had accepted you back in the program although I had to plead with them, vouch for you. Did you forget all that?"

Then I turned to Gloria, "Can't you do something about his attitude? This is going to cost him his dear life."

"His life is his," she replied. "He does whatever he feels like, has always been that way. All these trips to Tampa, to your office, to the hospital…it is taking a toll on both of us. I don't know how long I can handle him."

"Getting a new heart, going through that surgery, the drugs and care afterward—all look so difficult Doc. I am stressed out," Peter said. He was quite dejected.

"But smoking and boozing are not the answer," I said. "If you stop now, we can still get you into the program. It is not too late."

There were days when I felt like discharging him from my practice, but I knew that would result in his death right away. He needed round-the-clock attention. Once he even burst out in a loud fury, "It was your idea that I go for a cardiac transplant. Then they threw me out of the program. And now you want me to get back. What is the point? This is an emotional yo-yo!"

Looking back, I knew I had given more time and attention to this patient, but the thought that all those treatments and counseling were useless truly bothered me. Still I told him, "Calm down and go home now. Stay on the medications and don't touch one cigarette or a drop of booze. Maybe I could still convince Dr. McDaniel to reconsider, all right?" Gloria didn't appear to be happy. I gave him an appointment for one week and they departed.

August 2009

Again, they missed the next appointment. I was hoping they would call me soon, but nothing happened. Then I got a call from the ER.

"Your man is here again, this time in severe pulmonary edema. We are intubating him. Can you come to the ER right away?"

It was pandemonium in the ER by the time I got there. There was already a small crowd around Peter's bed. I could hear anxious voices all around as the doctor was shouting orders.

"Give me some epi, quick,

"Give me an amp of bicarb

"I need calcium.

"How are the pupils?"

"Oh, Doc, looks like it is flat line still."

He was already *coding*, with no pulse. The breathing machine seemed to be doing its job, but it didn't appear to be effective.

Somebody spotted me.

"Oh, here's Dr. Nathan. What do you want us to do? We have been coding him for almost fifteen minutes," the ER doc said.

"You can stop it now," I said. "I know Peter very well. He has been living on the edge, waiting for his cardiac transplant. No point in prolonging his agony. Let him go peacefully."

For a moment, my emotions got the better of me. Poor Peter had suffered enough. Although a lot of his misery was his own doing, I couldn't help myself feeling sorry for him as his life ebbed away right in front of me. And my own inability to pull him out of his miserable existence, a personal failure, gnawed at my mind. I felt angry at the transplant team for not accommodating him, but then I knew their hands were tied. For a moment, I felt mad at Peter for neglecting his own body and making his life as well as Gloria's a protracted agony. I guess that is what life is all about—you win some, you lose some. Every day, I see the ravages of my patients' errant behavior, resulting in so much morbidity and premature deaths, disruption of families, and more. Is there a solution in sight? I can't see anything in the foreseeable future. All I can do is keep trying to educate them in good patient behavior and hope they will comply with doctors' orders. Is that too much to ask from a patient who is on a suicidal path?[29]

[29] December 20, 2012

CHAPTER 30

Humor at the Office

In these days of high-tech medicine, demanding practice, electronic health records, etc., there is not much time left for listening to the stories of patients. But if you do make the time, the rewards can be great.

The world of medicine is a metaphor for emotions.

Hope and hopelessness, pain and joy, illness and recovery are all part of the landscape we live in. As you walk into your office or hospital every day, you don't know really what kind of situations you will face or experiences you will have. Some are very touching and poignant like the young parents who attend to their mentally retarded child with such love and affection that it will make you teary eyed. Others can be very funny like the woman who told me that she was light-headed as I walked into her room. Seeing the worried look on my face, she corrected herself, "Oh, I was just joking. I meant I am a blond." And still some others make you angry and irritable. Like the proverbial patient who calls you in the middle of the night for that nagging cough, which he had for several days, or the one who needs a refill of his medicines on Sunday morning.

Here are a few interesting situations that stand out in my memory.

Ruby

We often talk about compliance and why some patients don't get better in spite of seemingly good treatment. Some have a really good alibi. Here are a couple of examples.

Ruby came to the office complaining that she is still not feeling well and has a persistent headache. I took her BP which was significantly elevated. Lately her BP had become almost uncontrollable. "Let me look at the medicines. Maybe we need to change them a bit." I said. Ruby was a walking poly-pharmacy.

"Oh, I forgot to bring them," she said casually. That was the umpteenth time she had "forgotten"!

"Rubyyyy!" I said with a little fake annoyance in my tone.

"Oh, what is the big deal? I don't take them regularly anyway. I don't like these medicines," was her cool reply.

"Why? You didn't have any side effects. Besides they are lifesaving. You could have a stroke if you don't take your BP medicines regularly," I told her a bit strongly.

"You know, *St Petersburg Times* (our local newspaper) had a report on one of these drugs. It said the drugs are bad."

So, that is it. Yes, these days, the biggest medical journals are the local newspapers and patients trust them more than what their doctor recommends! Of course she had a good prescription plan and all. But still she didn't want to fill the prescriptions.

Now you know why some of your patients don't get better and develop many unwanted complications.

It took me a while to convince her of the necessity for proper drug therapy to control the hypertension. And I strongly advised her not to stop any medicines without checking with me. Often patients take the statements in the newspapers out of context if it suits them.

Roger

There are, of course, some patients who stop their medications when it is inconvenient for them. Roger has atrial fibrillation and is on Coumadin. He came for a follow-up. And his latest report of PT/INR was flagged in front of the chart. His INR was very low, suggesting he was probably not taking medicines as prescribed or had missed a few doses. He was beaming as I walked into the room.

"You look very happy, Roger," I greeted him.

"We are just back from a seven-day cruise. It was wonderful."

"That is good. How come your INR is so low? Did you eat too many veggies or miss some doses?"

The wife and husband looked at each other knowingly. And the wife said to her husband, "I told you, Roger, not to do it."

I raised my eyebrows.

Then Roger admitted apologetically, "You know, Doc, you told me that I shouldn't drink when I am on Coumadin. Right?"

"Right, yes, I said you can bleed from the stomach, you have to be cautious, especially when drinking liquors like whiskey, etc."

"But, there was so much wine and whiskey on the cruise, I decided to stop Coumadin for one week, so I could drink some. It was an all-inclusive fare, and I hated the wine to go to waste. I only stopped for one week. Is that too bad?"

John

John had been suffering from cancer of his larynx and already had a permanent tracheostomy after radical laryngeal surgery. He was also eighty-five, but relatively healthy looking in spite of all his serious problems. But he had been having intermittent dizzy spells, and one day he actually fainted.

On examination he appeared to have severe aortic stenosis, confirmed by further noninvasive studies.

So, I told him that he needed to undergo cardiac catheterization first and then consider fixing the problem with insertion of a brand-new valve. Yes, this would need open heart surgery. He immediately put his cylindrical metallic device on the tracheostomy hole in the neck and in a pitchless monotone said, "Doc, I don't want it."

"But you may get into serious problems with this. You can have sudden death."

"So be it. I am too old, I may die."

Now in came his wife. She also joined the debate.

"John, you should go through the surgery; you heard the doctor. Otherwise you can die,"

To which John answered in his robotic voice, "Why, you want your inheritance right away, dear?"

I decided it was better not to recommend the surgery. If I did, and he died, the wife would get away with not one but two inheritances, since the malpractice verdict would surely go in her favor.

Dorothy

Before I start examining a patient I spend the first minute asking about his or her family and what the patient has been up to since the last visit, etc., just to make the patient comfortable. When Dorothy Stevens came for her pacemaker checkup, I started with my usual question, "How is the family?"

Dorothy said she had a nice Christmas with her older daughter, Marina. But her twelve-year-old grandson was not quite well and threw a lot of temper tantrums after Marina's recent divorce. Now she was married to somebody twenty years older. "Oh, she threw the first one out," she said somewhat angrily.

"Why?" I asked.

"Oh, he was a pilot. He was cavorting with the pretty flight attendants. You know, when he goes on long flights to places like Caracas or Hawaii and so on. They have a stopover, and he must carry on with these pretty stewardesses. One day she confronted him. You know he had the audacity to say, 'Honey, I love you very much. But I like to date other women when I am away from home.'

"'Oh, really, now,' Marina asked him mockingly. 'You want an open marriage, right? No way, Jose, not on my life.'"

Then I started to talk about a book I had read recently, *Plane Insanity: A Flight Attendant's Tales of Sex, Rage, and Queasiness at 30,000 Feet*, by Elliott Hester, about the weird things that go on in the plane. Verbal arguments, demanding passengers, even sexual encounters! Economy passengers trying to sneak into first class cabins and hoping nobody would notice, things like that. We had a good laugh, and she left in a much better frame of mind.

In these days of high-tech medicine, demanding patients, and twelve-hour workdays, stuck in a dysfunctional health care system, we don't have much time for listening to these stories or reflections on daily happenings. But if you make the time, the rewards can be great. [30]

[30] Written during different times: 2000–2010.

CHAPTER 31

Curtain Call

In spite of detecting and correcting a pacemaker malfunction that may have saved the life, the patient was upset and left the practice. Everybody reacts to an adversity or a perceived adversity in a different way, the author found out.

Miriam K brought her sixty-seven-year-old husband, Jim to my office for evaluation of leg pains. It turned out that he did have significant peripheral vascular disease that was producing what doctors call claudication pains. He could walk no more than two blocks or so without pains.

The Doppler ultrasound studies of the legs clearly showed that he did indeed have major blockage in the main arteries in both legs. Being a chronic cigarette smoker and mildly diabetic, this was indeed what I expected.

"Looks like Jim needs surgery," I said. I showed her the results from the vascular lab.

"Oh, really," she was a bit surprised. But, I convinced her that the surgery is a must. Finally, he underwent femoro – popliteal bypass surgery (insertion of a Dacron graft that bypasses the block and restores the onward blood flow), first on the right side and then, on the left side. Both operations went well, but he had some post-operative complications that included a little infection in one area of the wound and an exacerbation of his chronic lung problems. They were all contained, and he recovered well and finally was home and started walking better.

During all the work up and admissions, I was very attentive to his problems and the wife was very happy about it. Miriam praised me fulsomely during the next several visits, often to my embarrassment.

One day, her family physician called me to see Miriam in the emergency room for recurrent syncope. Already suffering from hypertension and hypothyroidism, she had developed complete heart block, urgently needing a temporary pacemaker and subsequently a permanent one. For the next two years, I followed her pacemaker function diligently. When her family physician moved away, she adopted me as her primary-care doctor and cardiologist. Whenever I saw her, she was cloyingly pleasant.

Two years after the pacemaker implant, she had another bout of syncope while standing near her window. I immediately saw her in the office, and to my relief, the pacemaker checked out well. A Holter monitor did not reveal any pacemaker malfunction or significant arrhythmias of concern. The neurologist found nothing amiss, so I reassured her.

On another occasion, while adjusting the pleats on the window curtain, she fainted and woke up on the carpet. A neighbor brought her to the office. Again the pacemaker checked out well; it appeared to be pacing and sensing normally. A second Holter monitor was placed. When she returned the monitor, I asked her to wait at home for my call with the results. The monitor showed a pause of nearly three seconds with no pacer spikes. I grabbed the phone and called her right away but couldn't reach her. I was very concerned, "Maybe she has fainted and is lying unconscious in the house," I thought. So, I sent the local deputy sheriff to track her down. He found her in the neighbor's house chatting away and brought her to the ER.

I thought she would be pleased with all the hoopla and the special attention she got.

In the hospital, interestingly the pacemaker would stop functioning only when she raised her right hand over the head. Like she did while adjusting the pleats of the window curtains. That particular movement, it seemed, broke the pacemaker lead's contact.

From then on, the case was easy. The surgeon found a loose pin on one of the leads was intermittently disrupting the circuit. I congratulated myself and the pacemaker technologist for making the correct diagnosis and expected a double dose of praise from Miriam.

A few days later, she called my secretary and said:

"I am not coming back to Dr. Nathan's office."

"Why not? He fixed your pacemaker problem, didn't he?"

Instead of answering, she put the phone down.

"Looks like she is upset about something?" my secretary conveyed the message.

"Whatever for?" I was totally surprised at this turn of events. I thought I did an excellent job. Although I tried to call her several times it was of no avail. She wouldn't answer my call or return the messages. Soon afterward, I got a letter from a prominent trial attorney asking me to release her records. That took me by surprise. So, I asked my secretary to call her again. This time she opened up:

"I am upset, actually angry with Dr. Nathan for sending the police to take me to the ER. My neighbors were all looking at me when the police car showed up. I felt so small."

The lawyer obviously decided her allegation was groundless, so he proceeded no further.

I felt so sad that she was not concerned about her pacemaker malfunction that could have been fatal and the fact that after a good work up I was able to get to the bottom of the problem and actually fix it. This lack of gratitude was the last thing I expected from her, but I guess everybody reacts to an adversity or a perceived adversity in a different way. Fortunately, majority of my patients are grateful to my attention and treatment and that certainly make up for the small number who do not want to say 'Thank you.'

However I must also learn to embrace the concept, "Service is its own reward" as stated by Mahatma Gandhi.[31]

---

[31] A modified version was published in *Cortlandt Forum*, June 1998.

CHAPTER 32

Difficult Patients

Every doctor has to deal with difficult, demanding, noncompliant and sometimes arrogant patients in his or her practice. Instead of getting frustrated or angry one has to patiently understand them and develop one's own ways to handle them.

During the past many years of my cardiovascular practice, I have come across several difficult patients. They come in different personalities and attitudes. Some are pleasantly persistent while others are outright demanding. I have come up with my own classification of these problematic patients. I will illustrate them with one case each from my practice. They are indeed real cases, only the names changed.

Clever manipulator:

Dorothy is now fifty-five years old and suffers from coronary artery disease and insulin dependent diabetes mellitus. She had a coronary angioplasty about five years ago and did well for several months. Then she started getting chest pains. All out-patient work-up including a stress test and nuclear imaging were negative. She would call the office for emergency appointments or show up in the ER pleasantly insisting on admission. She used me and her family physician (FP) alternatively and on one of her numerous admissions with chest pains, her FP called me and asked,

"What do I do with Dorothy? Every time she is in the ER, she insists on being admitted. The (hospital) utilization committee is already after me, wanting her to be discharged."

"Well, let us go ahead and do a cardiac cath. This way we will know for sure if she has developed additional lesions or if the angioplasty is blocking?"

Next day, the cardiac catheterization showed patent angioplasty site and no major coronary occlusions. The findings were discussed with her, and she was reassured and discharged. But to no avail, a few days later she again appeared in the ER and this time it was her diabetes that was out of control.

I promptly admitted her and treated with IV Insulin drip and all the ancillary measures. Her blood sugars fluctuated a little and on two occasions blood sugars went down a bit resulting in some sweating and anxiety. She only had mild hypoglycemia. Finally she was ready to be discharged. That evening the nurse who was doing the accu-chek measurement of her glucose every six hours, said her blood sugar has shot up again. I told her to give some extra insulin. The following morning the nurse stopped me with this little information:

"You know Dorothy is always complaining of this or that and yet her appetite is good, and she walks around the floor without any sign of fatigue or discomfort, chatting with other patients. Her roommate told me privately that yesterday before I took her blood sugar with the accu-chek meter , she dipped her finger in the sugared coffee sitting on her table! No wonder she had a high blood sugar!"

"So, now we know why her diabetes is so labile," I said.

"She is a bit strange, isn't she!" the nurse added.

Dorothy is a divorcee and her daughter doesn't care for her much, and she is essentially a lonely soul. She wanted attention and some company, and she used the hospital more for her own recreation and support. Finally with a bit of counseling and a little help from social services, we were able to discharge her.

The annoying executive

Paul is a retired executive, from a large company and is the uncle of an Atlanta Cardiologist. In addition to an inquisitive mind, he has a questioning mind also and must know everything about everything related to his treatment. Sometimes quite overbearing, his visits to the office were quite time consuming. He must be in charge of everything including the conversation. However he liked me and always recommended my name to his friends. I patiently answered all his questions.

Paul suffered from Atrial Fibrillation that caused him frequent palpitations and Mitral Stenosis that gave him fatigue and shortness of breath. Finally he underwent a special procedure to dilate or enlarge his valve called balloon valvuloplasty. When I decided to start him on anticoagulant therapy, I had to talk to his doctor nephew. When I wanted to put him on digoxin to control his rapid heartbeats, "Can you check with my nephew please?" was his answer.

When he gets his monthly prothrombin time/INR to check the level of his anticoagulant therapy, I had to call him the same evening to discuss the results. I have given a standing instruction to all my patients that only if there is a change in dosage I will call them. That was applicable to everybody except Paul!

He would question the side effects of all drugs. And when he finally needed surgery for his valve and coronary artery disease, he wanted the angiograms to be done here but decided to go to Atlanta for the surgery. His nephew was there, so I couldn't object. And we carefully made copies of all echo studies and coronary arteriogram for him to take with him.

On one occasion my nurse, fed up with his antics, privately requested me, "He is a bit too demanding, isn't he? Maybe we should give him the pink slip?"

"Oh, we can't do that. He is a very educated person and hence very inquisitive. In a way that is good," I said.

Paul stayed with me for ten years and our relationship continued the same way. Age did not mellow him, he was always in charge, and I let him be. It seemed to work out well. Finally when he moved back to Atlanta to be closer to his nephew, he gave me a nice gift during his last visit in the office with a 'thank you' note.

Miss Noncompliant

Barbara worried me a lot. Both her husband and she were referred to me by a local family physician (FP), a good friend of mine, for cardiac evaluation and follow-up. Although she was not nasty or rude, she was always critical of almost anything she came across. She was also very strong-willed and pushy and quite opinionated. She had already seen two other cardiologists before. She suffered from severe hypertension and apparently couldn't tolerate many medications. Later I decided that she simply hated drugs and would exaggerate even trivial side effects.

"They tried to kill me," She said during her first visit.

"How so," I asked with some concern.

"Well, they tried to push all these drugs on me."

"But if you don't take them, you will be at high risk for heart attacks and strokes," I tried to remind her.

"Give me something else. I don't want any of these." She just waved a piece of paper with a long list of antihypertensive drugs. I glanced at it and almost burst into laughter. The list contained almost everything there was on the market! So during the next two months I went through all the other drugs she had not been treated with but it was of no use. She was "allergic" to them too!

Her husband, eighty years old, was seen by me for evaluation of chest pain. One day I brought him for a Thallium Stress Test. Actually Joe was a nice guy but clearly a hen-pecked husband. As soon as my technician was ready to get the signature for consent after detailed explanation of the test, she cut in, "You are not injecting that stuff into my husband."

Then I intervened, "Barbara, Thallium is an inert isotope. Nobody is allergic to that stuff."

Barbara was quite adamant and poor Joe looked at me helplessly. Finally I did the test without Thallium, knowing it will not yield complete results, just to appease the wife. Later I tried to gently nudge Barbara to see another cardiologist pointing out my inability to help her.

"Oh, I don't want to go to any other cardiologist. You are the third one I have seen and that is enough," she said emphatically. But she still wouldn't take most of the drugs I have prescribed. And her blood pressure always remained uncontrolled.

Both her family physician and I worried that one of these days, she will develop a stroke or heart attack, surely a malpractice waiting to happen. So I decided to formally discharge her from my practice, something I rarely do.

The dietitian who can't lose weight

Obesity is a common issue in our clinic and generates a lot of heated self-defensive discussion and at times some humor as well. What a patient fear most about me is my lecture on weight control, 'decalorification,' as I call it. Patients pretend they don't like my lecture but the spouses love it, especially if they are not overweight. And I promise them "If you lose at least one pound by the time you come for next follow-up, I won't lecture.'

So when Conrad, five feet ten, 325 pounds, came to see me, he had lost two pounds, and I congratulated him. Conrad has hypertension, diabetes, and mild heart failure. He steadfastly refuses to lose weight, and I suspect he eats everything in sight. When I try to teach him about dieting and exercise his answer is:

"You know, Doc, I know all about dieting, I was a dietitian for the school system before. This is just fluid. It is not fat. See here," and he lifted up the fatty tissue on his forearm and tried to convince me it is just fluid accumulation.

"Just give me some water pills. I will be all right," he added. Then I confronted him and explained why this was all fat and not fluid. Finally he admitted:

"OK, OK, I admit I *looove* food, what can I do?"

Next time he came in he had lost three pounds! I gave him a mock congratulation and asked:

"Hey, how did you do it?"

"Oh, I couldn't stand your lecture no more, so I didn't eat breakfast today and you promised you wouldn't lecture if I lost a pound.

"Well, I am glad you are on the right track. Can you then skip one meal every day?" I suggested.

"You want to know the real reason? My two grandchildren are with me now. They are twelve and fifteen. They raid the Frigidaire several times a day and gobble up everything in sight, so I don't have much to eat at home!"

So I suggested, "Maybe you should invite them to live with you permanently, what do you say?"

"Oh, no, Doc, I am trying to get rid of them somehow. They are not good for my wallet either."

The ultimate pet lover

Bill, suffers from COPD with bronchospasm, angina and already had a three-vessel CABG. But he is also in the ER almost every month with shortness of breath, and we are forced to admit him. He gets severe wheezing and usually responds to intravenous medications, inhalers, intense round the clock respiratory therapy etc. Within two days he gets better and wants to go home. Neither the pulmonary specialist nor I could find any real reason why he gets these frequent exacerbations. So one day I asked him: "Do you have any pets at home?"

"Yes, Dr. Nathan, I have a dog. He wanders in occasionally but mostly he stays outside," he said.

"So that may be why you are getting these wheezing episodes. You may be allergic to them, perhaps? Is there any possibility you can get rid of them" I suggested gently.

"OK, I will talk it over with my wife and will do so," he replied.

But to no avail. He continued his regular trips to the hospital and after a few visits, I decided to send the social worker to his house. Her report was interesting.

"Dr. Nathan, his house is worse than a pigsty."

"How, so?" I was curious.

"There are so many living under one roof...two cats, two dogs, several grandchildren who didn't look all that clean. And, the premises are so dirty, with a pile up of all kinds of trash, No wonder he gets asthma," she added.

"Oh, one more thing, I suspect he secretly smokes..."

During his next visit, I confronted him with all these new info and told him in no uncertain terms about getting rid of the pets, smoking cessation and cleaning the premises. He of course readily agreed but nothing really happened, and he continued his regular visits to the ER. And I told the pulmonary physician to take over the case although the patient wasn't happy about it.

As you can see these difficult patients come in all types. There is no question that every doctor has to confront difficult patients. Some can be very argumentative questioning your motives for every test and treatment, some can be vindictive and some others noncompliant with your treatment. It is rare that I have to give pink slip to anybody. Dealing with them is a real art that you learn from experience.[32]

---

[32] Written at different times 1998–2009.

CHAPTER 33

The Travails of a Traveler!

When you are a busy practitioner and time is of essence, the last thing you want is to experience delays and difficulties during your much-awaited vacation trip. But unfortunately air travel is not easy these days, the author found out.

It was a torrid Sunday; the thought of travelling even in an air-conditioned car made me uncomfortable.

"Hey, Delta called again. We have to be at Orlando airport at least three hours before check-in time," my wife mused.

"Why so early?"

"The security precautions, I guess. They have to check for bombs and what not, you know."

"Still, three hours is too much," I mumbled.

The thought of flying made me very skittish. After the TWA jet explosion and ValuJet crash and now the bombing in Olympic Village, I had become quite nervous. I had already had two brushes with death. First, it was a bicycle accident, while riding to the dorm in the medical school. I didn't see the car behind while turning. Then there was my kidney surgery, which was followed by multiple serious complications. Having survived all those, I wasn't quite eager to take any more risks. But how do you go to Mumbai, without boarding a plane?

"I have arranged a nice airport limousine to take us to the airport. It will be here, sharp at one o'clock. So be ready!" informed my wife.

"Looks like you have taken care of all the details! For once, I don't have to drive to the airport and look for a spot in the long-term parking garage. Today, we will travel in style." I was quite happy with the arrangements.

The limousine arrived promptly at 1:00 p.m. I took one look at the old worn-out taxicab and shouted, "This ain't a limousine!"

"Oh, don't worry, it will travel just as fast as the limousine." My wife was unfazed.

"I hope you are right."

The old driver came out and announced his name was Jerry. He obligingly carried the luggage from the doorstep to the trunk. It didn't quite fit into the trunk, so we had to use the backseat as well, drawing the ire of my teenage daughter.

"Ready to go to Tampa?" Jerry inquired.

"What do you mean? We are flying from Orlando International Airport. Didn't they tell you at the cab station?" I was quite perplexed. This trip was arranged almost a week ago.

"Well, they simply told me to take you guys to the airport. I assumed it was Tampa."

"No way!" Now my wife sounded angry. "I clearly told your manager where we were going, and he calculated the fare and all."

"I am the last-minute replacement. I don't even know how to get to Orlando airport." Jerry pretended his innocence.

"Well, that is nice to know. We will look at the map together." There was sarcasm in her voice.

"We will get there somehow." Jerry was reassuring.

The first thing we noted, after all three of us with the luggage squeezed into the car, was that there was very little air in the car. I started fanning myself with a newspaper.

"Well, I admit the AC isn't so great in this car. This is an old warhorse, you know. But it is pretty reliable." Jerry sounded somewhat apologetic.

Famous last words. My wife simply said, "I hope so," more in resignation. We started our trip and as we reached Tarrytown, about twenty miles from Brooksville and about-one third the way to Orlando, I heard a peculiar jolting sound from the left side of the car. Clearly the vehicle was quite unsteady and very wobbly. I looked at the driver knowingly, and he looked back. Anxiety was painted on his face. My wife tapped on my back. "Sounds like a flat tire, doesn't it?"

"Oh, no, not at this time," I said. I didn't even want to think about it. This would be a real fiasco.

"Well, we are having a slight tire problem." No sooner had he said it, there was mini explosion, announcing the suspected tire didn't work for us anymore! I was in total disbelief as to what was happening to a bunch of innocent travelers.

We drove a few more yards so that he could stop the car on a flat surface, and then stopped at a spot on a side road to change the tire. "This will only take a couple of minutes."

"It must be easy for you guys. You do this all the time, don't you." I was trying to reassure myself.

He went around and opened the trunk. He was simply standing there and looking somewhat puzzled. I sensed something very wrong. So I got out of the car and asked him.

"What do you know, I don't have a spare tire! Can you believe it?"

"No, I can't believe it. How come?" I was really losing patience. He simply stood there somewhat puzzled.

"How could you drive a taxi, without a spare tire?" I was totally mystified.

"Well, I know what you mean. But this is not even the car I drive normally." He sounded helpless.

I had talked with the company's manager only that morning, and they assured us that they would dispatch their best car and driver.

"Now, what we do? We are in a no-man's-land. I see only woods on either side for a long stretch," I said with anxiety.

"I guess we will slowly drive to the nearest gas station and phone." Which meant driving on the rim of the tire. There wasn't any more tire now. Suddenly I noticed that this car didn't have any radio phone.

"Oh, well, this is one of the old cars, you know," he said politely.

"You mean, the old reliable." Both of us laughed. Somehow we had gotten used to the idea that this drive was going to be a long one. Finally, we ambled along toward the nearest gas station about twenty yards up the road but the journey took almost twenty minutes. By the time we reached the gas station, even the rim had all but disappeared.

I was beginning to have second thoughts about this great vacation that I had been planning all year. After nearly two hours on the road, we hadn't cleared even twenty-five miles. At this rate when would I reach Mumbai?

We finally reached the gas station, and Jerry telephoned his company. He told us the replacement car and driver were on the way. It wouldn't be long now.

"Murphy's law is alive and well," my wife, ever the philosopher, proclaimed.

What do you know, in a few minutes, the new taxi with a young driver arrived, and we reached our destination in time to check in. I let out a long sigh of relief.

At Orlando airport, the queue for the international line of passengers was surprisingly light. Our passports were checked, and the security people asked a few simple questions. Satisfied that there were no bombs in our baggage, they let us proceed to the departure gate. We boarded the flight. Phew, we made it. Now I would safely reach my hometown in India.

Just before takeoff, the pilot announced that there was a problem with a valve that would not close automatically. The Frankfurt flight would be delayed by a half hour. Once in the air, the flight had no problems. Customs clearance in Bombay was a cinch, unlike the many times I had experienced during my previous flights. The officials were so polite that I could have cried!

We had a few hours to kill that night before we traveled to Cochin by Jet Airways. We took a room in Centaur, a posh hotel near Sahar Airport and enjoyed their sumptuous breakfast the following morning. That one-night stay cost me nearly $200—it was more expensive than the New York Hilton. We were not Air India passengers, that is why, I was told. The stay is free if you travel by Air India.

Our onward flight was scheduled for 9:45 a.m. We checked in at 9:00 a.m. What do you know, our flight was closed already. I just couldn't believe it. No amount of arguments could prevail. Although we were there a full forty-five minutes early, they couldn't fit us into their schedule, but we would be on the waiting list for the next flight. Anyway they put us on the next flight, which was going at 10:45 a.m. to Cochin. They gave us the green light to proceed to the gates. But while waiting in the lounge, a quick announcement came over the speakers: this flight is delayed because of bad weather in Cochin!

That was all I needed. I thought I was about to have a nervous breakdown. But it wouldn't do any good if I had one at that time. So I decided to postpone that event for a later time. Fortunately they announced that the rains had stopped in Cochin, there would be no more delay, and we could proceed to the aircraft. Wouldn't you know, it all turned out to be a blessing in disguise. Because of the torrential monsoon in Kerala, the first flight was diverted to Coimbatore and reached Cochin late, but our flight experienced no problems. And indeed our flight arrived earlier than the first flight. So I decided not to complain about this minor inconvenience.

Finally I landed in Cochin, my hometown, to the warm reception of friends and relatives who had assembled there braving the rains. I will always cherish that moment. They always gave me a reception fit enough for a king. They came in several cars to take me to my house and it looked like a mini motorcade. All of us then would sit down for a cup of coffee and some snacks mixed with small talk. Then I would take the lunch and dinner invitations from my relatives and friends, till my calendar was full. We tried to fit as much into our three weeks of vacation. This once-in-three-years pilgrimage to India really rejuvenates me.

I had already forgotten my problems of the flight and had accepted all those foibles as part of life.[33]

---

[33] August 2007

CHAPTER 34

Suddenly, Jaundice!

Beware of unapproved alternative therapies since they come with their own risks, as this patient found out.

Margot has been a regular in our weekly yoga class and has never missed a session. A champion ice skater during her younger days, she is very much a health-conscious person, sticking to a strict diet, exercising regularly, and taking nutritional supplements. Lean and toned, she looks almost a decade younger than her age of seventy-six. So it was surprising she didn't turn up for two classes in a row.

"What is the matter?" I asked her over the phone.

"Oh, you are not going to believe this. I have come down with severe jaundice!" she said.

"So far all tests are negative, can't find any cause," she added.

I sensed some fear in her words. I called Dr. Paul, her gastroenterologist, to get some details, with her permission.

"She clearly has painless, obstructive jaundice for sure," he said. "So far the abdominal ultrasound and CT scans of the liver, gallbladder, and pancreas are quite normal. Can't find a cause. No evidence of hepatitis. No gallstones. I went over her drugs; all she takes is a small dose of Lipitor for high cholesterol, which I have stopped already. But strangely, the jaundice hasn't improved."

Neither Dr. Paul nor I thought this small dose of Lipitor would produce such significant obstructive jaundice. Although Margot had lost only five pounds, this was noticeable on her thin frame. And she was beginning to look anxious and perturbed. Thoughts of cancer went through my mind, but I didn't tell her that. Also, all her scans had been negative, so where can the cancer hide?

"We are scheduling her for MRCP (magnetic resonance cholangio-pancreatogram) to make sure we are not missing any small tumors or polyps there," Dr. Paul added. This is a special imaging of the gallbladder, bile duct, and pancreatic ducts. It can reveal even a minor blockage in these areas that may have been missed in the previous studies.

After almost a week of outpatient work-up and wait-and-watch policy, no diagnosis was forthcoming. And jaundice persisted.

That was when Margot volunteered new information.

"You know, I go to an acupuncturist for my joint pains. And he suggested that I take these herbal preparations to boost my energy. I have been taking them for a while now. Do you think that would have anything to do with my condition?"

"Maybe," Dr. Paul replied optimistically. He asked her to stop the herbal supplements right away. He postponed the MRCP test and waited for a progress report.

Over the next two weeks, Margot's jaundice steadily improved, her itching abated, and she seemed to have more energy. After two more weeks, her jaundice had completely resolved, and she started coming to the yoga class. She proudly showed me her latest lab results—total bilirubin (a blood parameter for jaundice) had returned to normal levels, less than 1mg/dl! She was so happy that this turned out to be a benign condition with full recovery.

Later, I went over the herbal medicines Margot was taking and looked at the literature on the product. She took one pill each of Corydalis 5, a pain-relieving herb described in *Chinese Materia Medica*, along with Chang-Huo 13 for arthritis, and Bupleurum-Gardenia that is supposed to clear "heat" from various parts of the body. Interestingly, the latter is also recommended for viral hepatitis (to relieve jaundice presumably by reducing inflammation of liver cells!), to boost the immune system, vitalize blood circulation, and alleviate fatigue. She also took myrrh tablets for chronic inflammation and blood stasis. The Chinese acupuncturist told Margot these pills would improve her arthritis and fatigue, revitalize her body, and that her energy levels would increase.

She almost died taking them!

To say that more people are going beyond the borders of scientific medicine in search of a cure for their ailments or simply to improve and rejuvenate their health, is an understatement. Herbal supplements to boost one's energy and well-being have become all too popular. It has mushroomed into a multibillion-dollar industry.

Some of the commonly asked questions by my patients are:

"Can I take herbal medicines? They are natural, right?"

"Why should I take Lipitor? Doesn't garlic reduce cholesterol?"

"I just don't like drugs, period; can I try these supplements instead? They are harmless, I presume."

The manufacturers of these alternate health products often use catchy terms like "natural" (meaning it won't produce any harm), "energy booster" (implying it will enhance your overall performance), etc., and people often fall for these unsubstantiated claims. Which is one reason why there is a supplement boom in America. Not only have many of these products not held up well under scientific scrutiny, they can be outright harmful. Humans are always vulnerable, looking for magical cures for illnesses, influenced by appealing terms like "holistic health practice," "wellness revolution," "nutritional supplements to boost your immunity," "natural therapy," and so on. "Natural" doesn't always mean good for the body. In fact, some of the natural plant products could be potent poisons.

The commonly used Chinese herbs ginkgo biloba and ginseng can potentiate anticoagulants like warfarin, ephedra—containing herbal products used for weight loss—can cause hypertension and cardiac events. St. John's wort, given for depression, can interact with other antidepressants and antihypertensive medications. Most patients do not know that these products can be quite harmful and hence do not volunteer the information to their doctors. It is for this reason I ask new patients who come to my office if they are taking any supplements to boost their energy, reduce weight, etc. And I always tell them not to mix the allopathic medicines with alternative remedies without the explicit permission from their doctors.

Margot was lucky that she didn't have any long-term sequelae from this illness. But it could have been much worse.[34]

---

[34] November 2006

CHAPTER 35

The Doctor at the Other End of Stethoscope

A busy doctor never thinks that one day he or she can become sick and will have to put up with all the indignities and annoyances that the patients go through. The author learned a lot from the several episodes of illnesses that he had to suffer in his life.

Have you ever wondered how you would feel when you become sick like the rest of the patients you treat every day? Of course, when you are a young physician busy with your practice and family affairs, the thought that one day you would get old and infirm never crosses your mind, not to talk about the sudden unexpected problems that can crop up like what happened to me.

Health-related problems surfaced early enough in my life. First it was a case of severe amebic dysentery when I was only seven. I had to be carried physically to the neighboring hospital, a primary health center, on the shoulders of an able-bodied strong man whom my father hired, since there was no transportation in the remote island village where I grew up. That was for daily intramuscular injection of *emetine,* a drug given only in the hospital under a doctor's supervision.

Then at the age of eleven, while sitting in the classroom, the heavy black chalkboard, about 4' x 3', precariously mounted on a tripod and used by the teacher for writing, fell square on my head! I was sitting close to the board in my assigned seat on a bench waiting for the class to start when two students running around bumped into the board. I was too stunned to know what happened, but there was blood gushing from the crack on my scalp that eventually needed half a dozen stitches in the local hospital. Fortunately, I didn't suffer from any brain damage, but the hullaballoo that ensued was indeed very unpleasant.

In medical school I was constantly bothered with recurrent episodes of flu and missed a few classes, often bothered with allergies and urticaria and frequent conjunctivitis. I spent several days in the sick bay at the college hospital. But they were all minor compared to what would happen to me later in my life.

After graduation from medical school I proceeded to England for my graduate training in medicine. When I landed in London on February 5, 1965, it was snowing. The first time I ever saw snow! I almost wanted to go back home to my tropical abode in Kerala. Then there was the English food to reckon with. Such staples like roast beef and Yorkshire pudding, kippers for breakfast (!), and steak and kidney pie weren't exactly suited to my palate. They were a far cry from all the aromatic, spicy, mostly vegetarian dishes my mother cooked like *idli-sambar, dosa, mango pulisserry, thoran, dal vadai* (my all-time favorite), occasional mutton or shrimp curry, and more.

I happily joined Lodge Moor Hospital in Sheffield for my first job as a senior house officer, working in infectious diseases and internal medicine. Within three weeks, I came down with a severe case of chicken pox after taking care of a university student admitted with it earlier. Fortunately, I recovered without complications. Lying sick in the bed and being asked to follow the nurses' orders, the same nurses who had taken the orders from me the day before, was not much fun.

After completing my stint in England and passing all the required examinations to become a member of Royal College of Physicians of London (MRCP), a much-sought-after honor and a "must" for a consultant (attending) position in the UK or India, I went back to my home state Kerala in India but stayed there only for three years. I then decided to come to America, which would become my permanent residence for the rest of my life. After landing in America, it was smooth sailing for a while, although the winters in New York didn't agree with me, and I suffered from frequent respiratory infections and chronic bronchitis. So I moved to Florida, set up my practice, and was cruising well when the incredible happened.

I woke up one day with a severe headache. Not one prone to headaches even on a stressful day, I was puzzled. *Did an aneurysm blow up in my brain*, I wondered. *Or perhaps a vicious malignant tumor is growing in one of the cerebral hemispheres.* Doctors always think of the worst, you know that. It turned out that unbeknownst to me, my blood pressure (BP), so far normal, had shot up to 180/110! And that was the harbinger for a major kidney disease, *IGA nephropathy*! Not a single member of my family had suffered from kidney disease.

Next came a bad episode of angina, a heart attack, an angioplasty, a repeat angioplasty and stent, followed by allergy to morphine, resulting in severe vomiting of blood from an esophageal tear. Finally, things were settling. But not for long…my kidneys started failing.

"Ravi, you may need a transplant," Dr. P. M. Reddy, a good friend and my personal nephrologist, said without mincing words. I had always liked his approach, he is a straight arrow, telling me the truth the way it is.

"Oh, really!" I couldn't believe my ears. "Where am I going to get a kidney?" I wondered.

"Do you have any brothers or sisters who can donate one?" he asked.

I wasn't quite sure how you go about asking one of your siblings to donate a kidney. Suddenly it had become a burning issue. Fortunately one of my sisters was ready and willing, and so I brought her to the US.

Off I went to University of Minneapolis hospital for a kidney transplant. I couldn't thank my sister enough for her unique gift of life.

And on November 10, 1994, I received my precious transplant and got a new lease on life. That was only the beginning of the next cascade of problems. Another surgery on the second day to remove a big clot from the vein in the right leg, later a much-feared pulmonary embolism…then a period of calm. All was well till I got a heart attack ("My close call, your wake-up call" elsewhere in the book) that needed an emergency angioplasty and stent, and finally everything settled down.

Now I know what it is like to be at the other end of the stethoscope. How it feels like to be a patient and not a doctor. When you are healthy and on top of the world, belting out orders to nurses and techs, going from room to room examining patients, driving from hospital to hospital while listening to the audiotapes, taking care of the office affairs including the many problems that crop up frequently, you never think of all those ignominies your patients live through day in and day out. Walking around with backless gowns with nothing underneath, residents so junior to you coming to do the rectal exams, female nurses putting in a Foley catheter into the bladder, having to use a bedpan or bedside commode in the same ICU where you made your daily rounds…need I say more?

Then your friends come to visit you with flowers and fruits. And they look at you with sympathy. "Oh, you poor thing, how sorry we are for you…" Although they try to cheer you up with all the things you want to hear like, "You will be out of this place in no time," "The nurse said, you are already walking, that is great," etc, the words always ring hollow. Sometimes I doze off during the conversation from all the morphine, Demerol, and Ativan I am getting. When I open my eyes, they are gone. They have work to do; I can't blame them.

I know everything takes time, and I will also recover from this illness, I say to myself. There are millions of others suffering like me, but that is not much of a consolation either.

Hey, who said this life is easy?

But I never thought that I would have to go through such an obstacle course in life to reach where I am today. In any case, I am thrilled to be here to tell my stories. I have countless friends who were stricken at the peak of their careers and never lived to tell their story.

So, I guess I am very lucky. And I could retire having fulfilled my responsibilities and still have some time left to enjoy my two lovely grandchildren and one on the way. I am forever grateful to the Lord Almighty for His continued blessings.

What more can I ask for?[35]

---

[35] Brooksville, January 25, 2013.

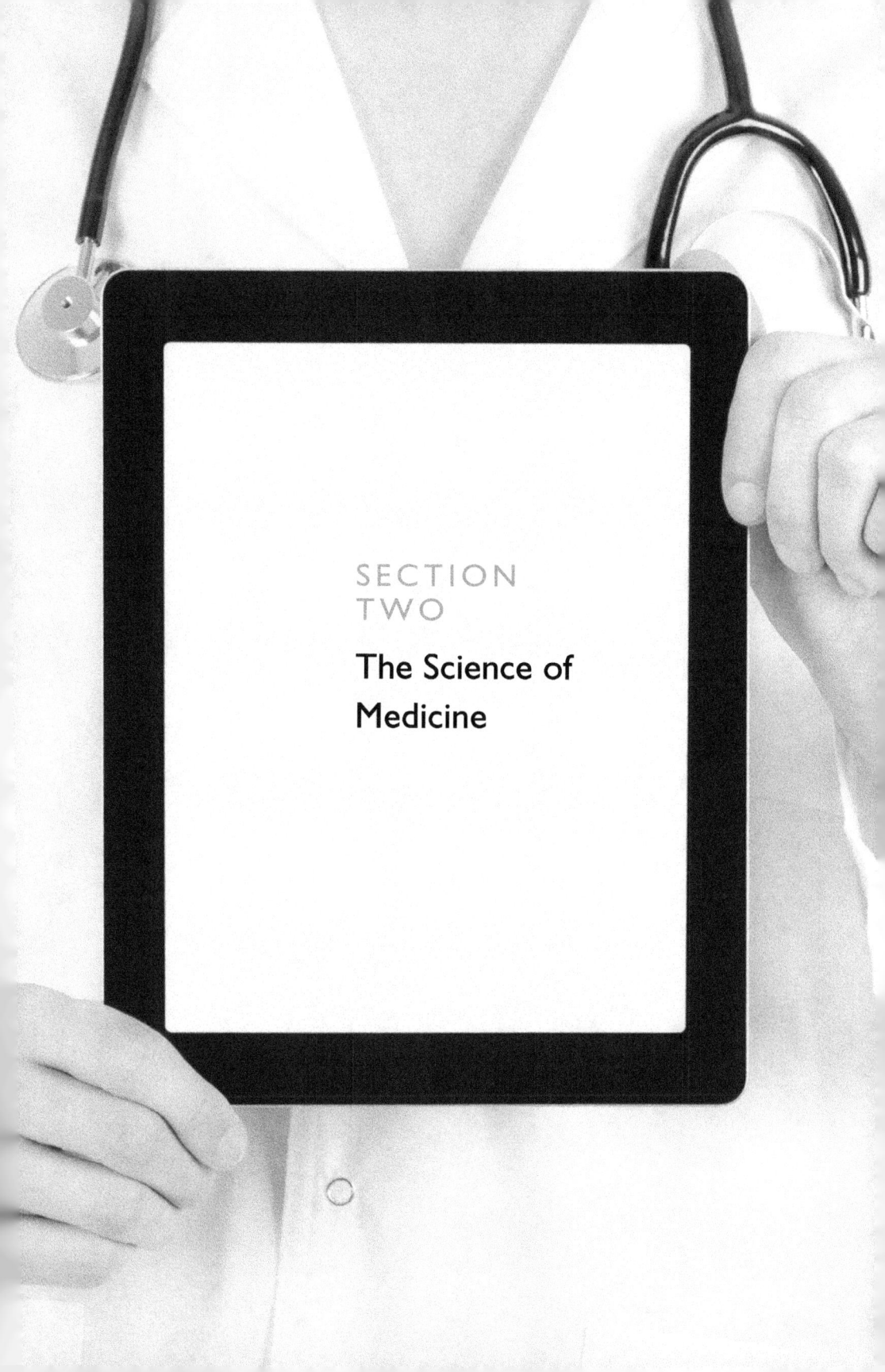

SECTION
TWO

The Science of Medicine

The Science of
Medicine

The greater our knowledge increases, the more our ignorance unfolds.

—John Fitzgerald Kennedy

When I was doing my cardiology fellowship in 1980, a patient who sustained a heart attack stayed in bed in CCU for more than a week, receiving precautionary intravenous medication to treat premature heartbeats. Blood thinners in any form were prohibited for fear of bleeding around the heart. Ultrasound and nuclear testing of the heart were primitive. There were few not-so-effective intravenous medications to treat a fast heart rate and no intravenous medications to treat chest pain, except morphine. Primitive pacemakers saved lives, but sometimes deteriorated the quality of life.

Fast forward to 2013. We get the patients out of bed as soon as possible after a heart attack. We don't give any routine intravenous medication to treat heart rhythm, as it was killing the patients. We take them to the cath lab and open the blocked blood vessels within an hour or two, using many different blood thinners, as the mainstay of treatment. We now have several choices of intravenous medications, which work instantaneously, to treat fast heart and chest pain.

We have many types of pacemakers and even implantable defibrillators not only to treat a slow heart, fast heart, and heart failure, but also to prevent sudden cardiac death.

Now, we have of three-dimensional and four-dimensional ultra-sounds, nuclear scans, MRI, and electrical mapping to study the heart. We almost replaced open heart surgery and carotid artery surgery, using stents to treat symptoms from clogged blood vessels and also for treatment of aneurysms. And for those who have sustained irreparable damage of the heart, cardiac transplantation is a viable option.

We started with stem cell therapy and are advancing to cell therapy without cells. "Genomics, proteomics, metabolomics, and nanomedicine," the words that were never heard until recently, will bring new advances for therapy in the near future and renewed hope for diseases once thought to be untreatable.

Some of the stories in this book illustrate how these medical advances have come to the rescue of the critically ill patients who otherwise may have lost their lives or become quite disabled from the sheer extent of their illnesses.

However one word of caution. Even though the technological advances are expanding exponentially, the passion for medicine and compassion for people—so evident in Dr. Nathan's personal stories—is slowly becoming a scarce commodity in real practice. The healing power of simple words and a tender touch is gradually becoming a lost art.

"The good doctor treats the disease; the great doctor treats the patient with a disease," said Sir William Osler, one of the greatest physicians in history. What a true and profound statement. We have to wait for the pendulum to swing back, to enjoy the best of both worlds.

Rao Musunuru, MD, FACC, FAHA, FCCP
Chief of Cardiology, Bayonet Point Medical Center, Hudson, Florida
National Physician of the Year award from the American Heart Association 2005
Medical Columnist, *Tampa Tribune* and *Tampa Bay Times*

CHAPTER 36

My Close Call, Your Wake-Up Call

I was a workaholic, never realizing that long hours were chipping away at my health.

A little chest tightness nagged at me as I finished my work out on the treadmill. It worsened while I was in the shower, but still no radiation of pain or diaphoresis. My physician wife, Susheela, insisted on a stat ECG anyway.

I should be all right, I told myself. In any event, I couldn't afford to get sick on a Tuesday; Tuesdays are quite busy for me.

But all hell broke loose at the Emergency Department (ED). My chest pain intensified despite a sublingual nitro and IV analgesics. I became diaphoretic and felt the typical jaw pain. I knew too well what it felt like because I'd experienced it ten years ago during my first episode of angina.

When I became dizzy, I asked the ED doctor to immediately contact the senior cardiologist, a friend of mine. He and his partner came just in time. The pain had become unbearable. Cold sweat enveloped me. I peeked at the cardiac monitor and couldn't believe what I saw, some early ischemia. This was the last thing I expected. I thought I was doing well. I'd become obsessed with diet and exercise since my first cardiac episode, and I took my medications regularly.

The next few hours are foggy. I could hear urgent voices and concerned whispers.

"Morphine." "No! No! He's allergic. Give Demerol instead."

"His heart rate is 40, pressure dropping…He's in cardiogenic shock!"

"How many IV sites do we have? Rush fluids. Get him an amp of atropine!"

"Administer TNK?" "Oh, he's on warfarin? OK, heparin."

"Contact the Hudson Heart Institute, stat." That was the tremulous but firm voice of Susheela, my wife. It was exactly what I would have said, had I been able.

"What about BUN and creatinine?" My question exactly. Since my renal transplant, the possibility of my kidney failing now made me shudder.

Could I be dying? If not, would I have to live the rest of my life as a cardiac cripple? Would I forever be dependent on my wife and kids?

My colleagues worked on me feverishly during the next hour. They started IV Integrilin and alerted the cath lab at the Hudson Heart Institute. As I was lifted into an ambulance, my consciousness faded. I learned the rest of the story from my wife.

I'd been wheeled straight to the cath lab. My blood pressure was 70 mmHg systolic, pulse 55. My right coronary artery had acutely occluded at a proximal location. The interventional cardiologist and his team opened two blockages and placed stents. The response was dramatic.

I awakened slowly and saw the faces of my anxious wife, two smiling cardiologists, a cardiac surgeon, a few of my friends, and some nurses. No chest pain!

"What happened? Where am I?" I asked tentatively.

"The emergency angioplasty is over. You're fine," Susheela said, visibly relieved.

"You're fine now," the cardiologist reassured me. "But, you cut it too close." Later he told me he thought he'd lost me. I'd stopped breathing, and he thought he couldn't get the wire in fast enough.

I had that sense of impending doom experienced by most heart attack patients. My electrocardiogram showed evidence of a heart attack in the back wall of the heart called inferior myocardial infarction (IMI). The storm had subsided, and I'd made it safely to the shore—for now.

The cardiologist speculated on my IMI's likely etiology.

"Probably a plaque rupture. No one knows why. Your lipids are good, BP's under control. Could be stress-related—all that catecholamine release."

How close was my brush with death? Since then I've had time to wonder what's happening to the health of doctors in general. A fifty-seven-year-old physician friend of mine recently died in his sleep of cardiac causes. Another of my colleagues, only forty-seven, had an acute myocardial infarction and was saved by angioplasty. Yet another friend, fifty-three, just underwent a triple bypass. Doctors are clearly under a lot of stress. We have no time to take care of ourselves. Or we don't make the time.

My heart attack episode was last spring. I've resumed my practice, but on a much lighter schedule. I've scaled down my pace of life. I now do yoga and play with my cat and smell the roses with my wife.

On my first day back, patients greeted me with, "You have to take care of yourself. We need you." And that's exactly what I plan to do: be there for those who need me.

My heart attack made me realize that life happens in the present. Every day now I live in conscious appreciation of the gift of life.[36]

[36] Reprinted with permission from *Medical Economics*: June 4, 2004; 81:42, 44-44. *Medical Economics* is a copyrighted publication of Advanstar Communications, Inc. All rights reserved.

CHAPTER 37

Second Chance: The Story of a Cardiac Transplant

Cardiac transplantation has come of age. That is the good news. But finding a suitable donor heart is the hardest part.

When Bradley Stone walked into my office one day, he looked almost the symbol of health: tall, chubby-faced, with a baritone voice, and a full lock of hair on the top, slightly graying at the temples. Having retired to Florida at the age of fifty-five years, he wanted to establish with a cardiologist first and then pursue his favorite sport of golf.

Brad had his first heart attack at the age of forty-two while working as an insurance executive in Buffalo, New York. Fortunately, heart catheterization showed only a minor blockage in one of the coronary arteries and mild damage to the heart muscle. He was relieved when told that he wouldn't need any bypass surgery. He changed his lifestyle, cut out the sausage and eggs from breakfast, steaks from dinner, gave up cigarettes altogether, and, with some difficulty shed the excess flab. He thinned down from 220 pounds to 180 and looked fitter than ever.

Brad enjoyed two glasses of wine before supper. It was the doctor's orders to raise his "good cholesterol" and prevent further blockage in the coronary arteries! At least that was his reasoning. I suspected that he was drinking more but didn't probe him any further.

During the next few years, Brad regained most of the weight back that he had lost with careful dieting. Then one day he landed in the emergency room with shortness of breath. He was told that he had developed heart failure and his heart muscle had some damage; it was better that he quit working and retire to Florida. That was when he established with my practice.

I saw him periodically, and with strict diet, some exercise, and occasional adjustment of medications, Brad did quite well, his heart failure seemingly under control. We became good friends as well; it wasn't the usual doctor-patient relationship anymore. He talked to me about his new golf buddies at the Brooksville country club and volunteer work at the local church while I would talk about Hindu philosophy like meditation, vegetarianism, etc., to improve the healing process. We had other common ground as well, like my son entering the Boston University School of Medicine whereas his nephew was graduating from the School of Medicine at University of Virginia.

I didn't see him for a while, and he may have missed an appointment or two. I presumed he was doing quite well; otherwise, he would have called me. Then suddenly one day he showed up, barely able to breathe, and I had to rush him to the intensive care unit. With intravenous diuretics and deft ICU handling, he regained his breath and felt better. But I knew that something really had gone awry this time.

A few tests, including a cardiac ultrasound and heart catheterization, made the diagnosis clear. Brad had developed a condition called dilated cardiomyopathy that resulted in an enlarged and flabby heart with poor pumping function. This caused a backup of fluids in the lungs that made breathing quite difficult. Although one could tone up a failing heart with drugs, the long-term prognosis was poor and sooner or later he would succumb to his disease. During the next few weeks it became painfully obvious that my dear friend was slowly deteriorating and often couldn't execute simple functions without stopping to catch his breath. A repeat echocardiogram had shown significant deterioration of his left ventricular function.

I decided to have a conference with Brad's entire family. His nephew, a doctor, knew the seriousness of the situation.

"Brad's heart is not getting any stronger in spite of all the good drugs. He is retaining more fluid," I summarized the problem. "He will be back in the hospital soon," I reluctantly added. I didn't quite have the heart to tell them that this diagnosis was tantamount to a death sentence. It was just a matter of time.

"Can't you do anything more? Brad was so full of hope when we moved and was looking forward to his life in Florida," Diane, his wife, said with great concern. "He is only sixty-three, you know," she said. I certainly agreed that he was relatively young to give up hope for long-term survival especially in this era of dramatic advances in medical sciences.

"Well, he needs a new heart...I mean a cardiac transplantation," I finally forced the words out of my mouth.

"Really...!" Both Brad and Diane were speechless for a moment. When they gained composure, Diane asked, "Heart transplantation, huh? I thought you were joking. Is that possible?" Diane still had that incredulous look on her face. She didn't think it was an attainable goal for her husband.

"Yes, it is very much a viable treatment now. As a matter of fact, Tampa General Hospital has done more than 150 of them successfully. The head of the cardiac transplantation program, Dr. Vijay, is a good friend of mine." I tried to sound confident. I had to keep his hopes up.

I could sense that both Brad and Diane were still uncomfortable with the idea. I tried to figure out what was going through their minds. The heart has always been the symbol of love and life. It is where your soul resides; well, at least that is the belief. It has spiritual and religious significance. Most people cannot even conceive of the idea of replacing that marvelous organ. That is why, when the first heart transplant was done in South Africa by Prof. Christian Barnard, it captivated the attention of the entire world.

"Don't you think Brad is a little old for this? He is not a young man, you know," Diane said after a few minutes of silence. They were worried whether Brad could make it out of the operating room after what would be a dramatic and complex surgery.

"In Tampa, they transplant hearts up to sixty-five. One thing in favor of Brad is that the rest of his body appears to be healthy. Anyway this is his only chance," I tried to reassure them. I had to somehow make them accept the idea of replacing his heart. I knew in my heart that it would be a formidable surgery, especially for a very sick man like Brad. Moreover, he would be on lifelong treatment with drugs to prevent rejection of the new organ. I discussed briefly the current high success rate in cardiac transplantation and the many advances medical science has made in this regard.

"Of course everything depends on the availability of a donor heart. Unfortunately many more patients are waiting than there are donor hearts available for transplantation." I tried to put everything in perspective. Finally they gave me the green light.

The first step was to contact the transplant coordinator, Jane Stevenson, at Tampa General Hospital. She was very happy to arrange for the preliminary transplant workup, which included a plethora of tests like cardiac biopsy, HLA matching, psychiatric evaluation, just to name a few. For Brad it was an exhausting five-day stay in the hospital. There was unanimous agreement that he would need a new heart soon. He was perennially short of breath and often forgetful too, an effect of lack of oxygen in the brain. The transplant team was concerned about his wine indulgence although Brad had been dry for at least a year now. They obviously didn't want the new organ to fall apart because of his booze.

"We will submit Brad's case to the transplant committee for discussion and approval," said Jane after reviewing all the records. I fervently vouched for his mental stability, family support, compliance with medical treatment, etc., in an effort to convince them that he was certainly worthy of a transplant. On the day when his case was discussed by the transplant panel both Brad's family and I were quite nervous. And our joy knew no bounds when Diane called me with the good news that Brad had been accepted for transplant. *Well, the first hurdle is over*, I told myself. I knew there would be many more before a successful transplant was accomplished.

Now the waiting game began. First Brad's name was added to the list in the computer organ matching program, a national network called UNOS. That meant Brad would be eligible to receive a donor heart from anywhere in America. Brad knew that the donor organ would have to be matched with his blood group, HLA antigens, body size, and so on. He knew the usual waiting period to get a donor heart would be anything from eight months to infinity. Frankly I was not sure whether he could make it longer than a few weeks. In fact, my first referral, Billy Clemens, a few years ago, died at the age of fifty-seven while waiting for a transplant. Since then, I have been painfully aware that too many people die with their hopes never realized. I quickly stamped out such negative thoughts from my mind.

He came back to Brooksville with renewed energy and hope for the future. He also showed me his new beeper, which made it easy for the transplant team to page him at all times, when a donor heart became available. He was ready. As for myself, I ceased to be his doctor; instead, I became part of his family...anxiously waiting.

But it was not going to be that easy. One day I got a call from the emergency room. It was Brad again, his third admission in less than three months. He was in pulmonary edema and this time it was a very close call. We pumped out all the fluid from his lungs. His heart had to be supported by special medications and, when he was discharged, I arranged a home health care team to give him daily intravenous medicines to tone up his weak heart. He even had a permanent catheter called an infusaport inserted into the subclavian vein below the left clavicle, for ready venous access.

Brad was hanging by a thread...barely.

"How long can I continue like this?" he asked me after his last admission. The fear of early death was clearly reflected in his eyes. I knew he was walking on eggshells.

"I don't know, Brad. We are doing everything we can to keep you going. Who knows, Tampa General may call you with a heart tomorrow." I wanted to keep his hopes high. But I knew any minute now, the heart could stop, and he would move into eternity just like Billy Clemens. Was history going to repeat itself?

Later Diane asked me privately, "Brad is not going to make it, is he?"

"Don't even think about it." I didn't know what else to say. "It all depends on if he can get a heart soon enough," I added since I didn't want to give her any false hope.

No call came from Tampa for the next several days and Brad was getting dejected. I was too. I was losing heart realizing that Brad wouldn't be with us very long if he didn't get a heart soon enough. During each hospitalization, in panic myself, I personally called the transplant team and apprised them of his urgent need. At one point while admitted to the ICU, his pressure was so low, I thought he wouldn't survive that night. The end was in sight and it was frightening. I had never felt this close to a patient. I simply didn't think that I could carry him anymore on my shoulders. I called Jane to see if Brad's name had moved up in the computer.

"He will get the top priority now," Jane tried to reassure me. "But as you know, hearts are difficult to come by." She sounded helpless.

On July 2, 1994, I got a call from Phyllis, Brad's doting sister. "Hey, they have a heart for Brad. We are on our way to Tampa General Hospital," I was thrilled; finally a heart for the dying man. It couldn't have come a moment too soon.

"Is he afraid to go through the surgery?" I asked Phyllis, although I knew the answer.

"Are you kidding? He knows this is his last chance," Phyllis was almost exuberant. "Brad was praying for this moment."

Brad went into surgery about 4:45 a.m. Somewhere in Fort Myers, there was a car crash and an eighteen-year-old boy died. He was a perfect match for Brad. One of the cardiac surgeons took off quickly in a helicopter and did the harvesting surgery. He removed the donor heart, put it in an ice-filled cooler, and rushed back to Tampa General Hospital. By that time Brad was already under anesthesia and his chest was being opened by another surgeon. Excellent timing and coordination, I said to myself. The surgery went without a hitch.

I let out a big sigh of relief and happiness.

Immediately after surgery, heavy doses of cyclosporine and prednisone were started to prevent rejection, a much-dreaded complication with all transplants. He came off the respirator smoothly. For the first time, Brad could really breathe easy. His courage and determination finally paid off. Diane was jubilant. She didn't think that she would ever see this day.

Then came a few setbacks. Two days later, Brad couldn't see through his right eye. He felt that his left arm and leg had become a little weak. He was very perturbed.

"Now what is the matter? I have a good heart but why can't I move my arm?" he asked. He was quite anxious.

The neurologist patiently explained that he had developed a mild stroke and not to worry for the moment. With physical therapy, indeed he felt better. But soon he suffered his first bout of rejection, a dreaded complication with organ transplantation. A diagnostic biopsy of the new heart showed early signs of rejection. His antirejection drugs were revamped, new drugs added, and finally the problem was controlled. Later he developed a skin rash from a drug allergy. That turned out to be a minor problem when compared to the depression he sank into soon.

Finally, after a twenty-day hospital stay, Brad came home with a smile on his face. I put him through our cardiac rehabilitation program where he was considered a hero of some sort, and he certainly was the center of attention. Six months later he was hanging out on the golf course, flaunting his new heart.

Now that Brad has celebrated the anniversary of his transplant, he is wearing his "gift of life" with great pride and gratitude. He has a lot more hair on his head that is darker and healthier.

"Hey, I can go to bed every night without the fear of waking up gasping for air in the wee hours of morning," he said with a sense of relief. He can't believe this transformation. His only complaint now is, "If I have an eighteen-year-old heart, why can't I 'perform' like an eighteen-year-old"? Diane blushes a little and gently prods his back every time he pops the question.

Cardiac transplantation has come of age. That is the good news. But finding a suitable donor heart is the hardest part. "A lot of people are waiting for one; they are in short supply. We just happened to be lucky," said the surgeon later.

A surge of satisfaction warms up my whole body and mind, just watching the victory of science over death.[37]

---

[37] Reprinted with permission from St. Petersburg Times: Heart Transplantation gives hope to patients: St. Petersburg Times/ Hernando Times: Friday, Feb 2, 2001.

CHAPTER 38

A Catastrophic Pulmonary Edema from Nowhere

Since medical errors are being reported frequently these days we need to make absolutely certain that no adverse consequences occur during any diagnostic or therapeutic procedures because of an oversight on the part of medical staff.

One Saturday just as I was going for a lunch break, a "routine" cardiac consult was called in on a patient who was admitted the day before.

"What is the problem, Rosy?" I asked my nurse who took the call. Although it was called in as routine, sometimes these cases have a way of turning seriously ill all too quickly and hence I don't like to take any chances. By the time I finish at my office and do all the paperwork, it could be late evening.

First a little background on the patient. Mr. Summers, seventy-six years old, whom I had known for many years, suffered from a lot of medical problems including chronic heart failure (HF) and chronic lung disease, COPD in medical parlance, obviously from his long history of smoking,. A few years ago, he developed cancer of the prostate gland that was treated with radioactive seed implants and had been disease-free. Eight years ago he had an acute heart attack that needed a four-vessel coronary artery bypass surgery (CABG).

He remained well for about five years and then started experiencing intermittent exacerbations of his COPD. This seemed to precipitate recurrent bouts of HF, needing a few hospitalizations. An ultrasound study of the heart showed that the effective pumping fraction (ejection fraction, or EF) was down to almost half of what it should be, about 30 percent only (normal being 55–75 percent) Although with medical treatment, his health remained stable, and I was cautiously optimistic about the long-term prognosis.

A heart catheterization was done a year ago during one of his admissions with chest pain. And it showed that all his bypass grafts were patent. Only a small coronary artery branch had some narrowing but that didn't warrant any intervention. However his EF had deteriorated significantly to just about 20 percent. Although treated conservatively with medicines with some initial improvement, he started having more problems. He had to be admitted again for palpitations and dizziness that turned out to be from a dangerous form of heart rhythm disorder known as ventricular tachycardia. Then he had an episode of ventricular fibrillation a lethal arrhythmia if not treated promptly. This warranted insertion of a pacemaker and an automatic defibrillator that would correct the abnormal rhythm with a gentle electric shock.

As if all these complications were not enough, Mr. Summers also had a bout of pneumonia from which he recovered with difficulty. He had suffered from mild chronic anemia, most likely due to a combination of his bleeding peptic ulcers, chronic rheumatoid arthritis on *methotrexate* therapy, and chronic diverticulitis. I saw him just three weeks prior to this admission in the office. His HF was under very good control, and he had lost some of his excess weight too.

The current admission was primarily for his abdominal pain, possible gastrointestinal (GI) bleed, and anemia. Because of his cardiac history the family physician wanted me to look in on him while he was undergoing GI workup and emphasized that his cardiac status was quite stable.

As I leisurely walked into his room I saw an incredible scene—he was gasping for air! The nurses and technicians were crowded around him, some adjusting his nasal cannula delivering oxygen, others pushing medicines. The monitor tech said that he was trying to contact me.

He was obviously very short of breath, ashen pale, sweating profusely, and in acute distress. He was breathing faster, his heart rate had gone up, and BP had dropped to 95/70 mm of Hg. His neck veins were visibly engorged and standing quite prominent, a sign of pressure buildup inside the heart.

I took my stethoscope and listened to his chest. His lungs were rattling away, and I could hear a lot of wet sounds called *rales* throughout both lung fields. On listening to his heart a faint murmur and an extra sound were audible, what we call gallop rhythm, probably indicating that a valve may be leaking and the heart is under strain. A pulse oximetry revealed that his blood oxygen saturation had dropped to 65 percent even on high flow oxygen! This was indeed quite low, suggesting the patient was in a crisis.

When I turned around, I saw the wife approaching me in a state of panic. "What is going on, Doctor? He was OK just half hour ago," she said.

"I don't know exactly, but I will find out right away," I promised. "All I can tell you is that he has gone into pulmonary edema," I added. Then I said to the nurse, "Tell me what happened."

"Patient was fine when he left for the CT but seems to have taken a turn for the worse after he returned. I asked them to page you."

It was clear that he had developed an acute pulmonary edema. A quick portable chest X-ray showed both lungs were full of large fluffy infiltrates, typical of severe bilateral pulmonary edema, in sharp contrast to the relatively clear lung fields in the X-ray taken the day before. The radiology technician vouched that the patient left the department in good condition. When asked about how much dye he received for the scan he said, 110 ccs of Isovue 300,—a nonionic radio-opaque contrast media. Nonionic dyes are supposedly safer.

"Isn't that a lot of dye?" the nurse asked. I also had the same question since our cardiac procedures generally needed only about 50 ccs or less.

Mr. Summers was clearly in severe distress because his lungs were over-loaded with fluid and secretions. He was drowning in his own secretions that clogged up the air passages and warranted aggressive therapy. The nurse had already started him on oxygen with a nasal cannula but that wasn't sufficient.

Time was of the essence. I quickly barked some orders to the nurse, all in quick succession.

"Give him IV Lasix and some morphine."

"Where is the oxygen mask? This nasal cannula is not sufficient."

"Call the RT. He needs a breathing treatment."

"Get a bed in the ICU. Need to transfer him quickly. We may have to intubate him."

"Insert a Foley catheter, let us see if he is making urine."

After giving some of these emergency measures, he stabilized a little and was transferred to the intensive care unit, with preparations being made for intubation and ventilatory support. He rallied well with large amounts of intravenous Lasix, a powerful diuretic, along with 100 per-cent oxygen by mask, a small dose of IV morphine,,and lots breathing treatment.

On review of the charts, it appeared that he had significant anemia on this admission that had improved with just one unit of packed red blood cell transfusion. He was able to tolerate that amount of fluid in his sys-tem. There was no sign of infection like a pneumonia to account for the current deterioration. Subsequent workup showed a slight elevation of an enzyme called *troponin* to 4.1, suggesting he may have suffered a small heart attack but there were no changes in his EKG to suggest that he was actually having a heart attack. A quick ultrasound of the heart also failed to show any new changes, suggesting he didn't have any permanent insult to his heart.

Mr. Summers continued to improve under proper therapy and was eventually released from the hospital. Six months after this episode, he remained well with good control of HF.

So what really happened to our patient? In order for us to understand the dramatic onset of HF within a few minutes after intravascular administration of a radio-opaque contrast media, we needed to know the physiological and pharmacological effect of the dye that was injected for contrast imaging while doing a CT scan.

The sequence of events suggested a causal connection in a patient who has preexisting cardiac dysfunction. One could argue that he may have suffered a spontaneous heart attack that precipitated this catastrophic pulmonary edema but it seemed less likely because of the close proximity of the event to the time of injection of contrast medium and his stable cardiac status prior to admission. The other possibility was that he could have had a sudden allergic reaction, although there was no history of such a reaction in the past. A third possibility, most likely in this case, was an exaggerated physiological effect in a patient with compromised heart.

Radio-opaque dyes are hyperosmolar compounds and will increase intravascular volume. Osmolarity by definition is "a measure of the osmotic pressure exerted by a solution across a semipermeable membrane (one that allows free passage of water and completely prevents movement of solute) compared to pure water."

Isovue, given to our patient, is nonionic with low osmolarity of 616 (mOsm/kg water) compared to previously used agents like Renografin, which has a much higher osmolarity of 1450. Still, it is higher than that of blood, which has an osmolarity of 300. So, when the dye is injected into the blood, the osmolarity of blood goes up, and it would start sucking fluids from the tissues, which it wouldn't in the normal status. This transient osmotic circulatory volume overload dumps fluid into the lung, leading to pulmonary edema, as happened in this case. The development of such decompensation is related to the volume and speed of injection, size of the vein used, underlying kidney problems (if kidneys are not functioning well, then they may not be able to clear the excess fluid in the body in the form of urine), and the general health of heart and lungs.

After we started using nonionic contrast like Isovue few years ago, we haven't seen any acute pulmonary edema resulting from its usage in our hospital. But cases like this are reminders that such complications occur, and hence it is important to document the adverse event in the patient chart. There is a burgeoning elderly population all over the globe, especially in the US with heart muscle weakness resulting from coronary heart disease. They also have varying degrees of heart failure and in these patients with compromised cardiac function and often mild kidney insufficiency even a small amount of dye can increase the osmotic pressure in the blood and tilt the balance toward heart failure and pulmonary edema.

Scientific advances over the past few decades have been phenomenal and have helped us to diagnose and treat our patients effectively. However they all come with a price. Some of these new tests and treatments are not without danger. In this case, as in most other cases, a modest dose of 50 cc of IV contrast during the CT scan would have been enough to get the necessary information. Any patient, especially if there is a history of heart disease, should be closely observed for several hours following contrast injection to avoid a catastrophic pulmonary edema. In this day and age when medical errors are becoming frequent, often resulting in deaths, we need to make absolutely certain that no adverse consequences occur during any procedure because of an oversight on the part of medical staff.[38]

---

[38] A modified version was first published in *Cortlandt Forum*, July 2005.

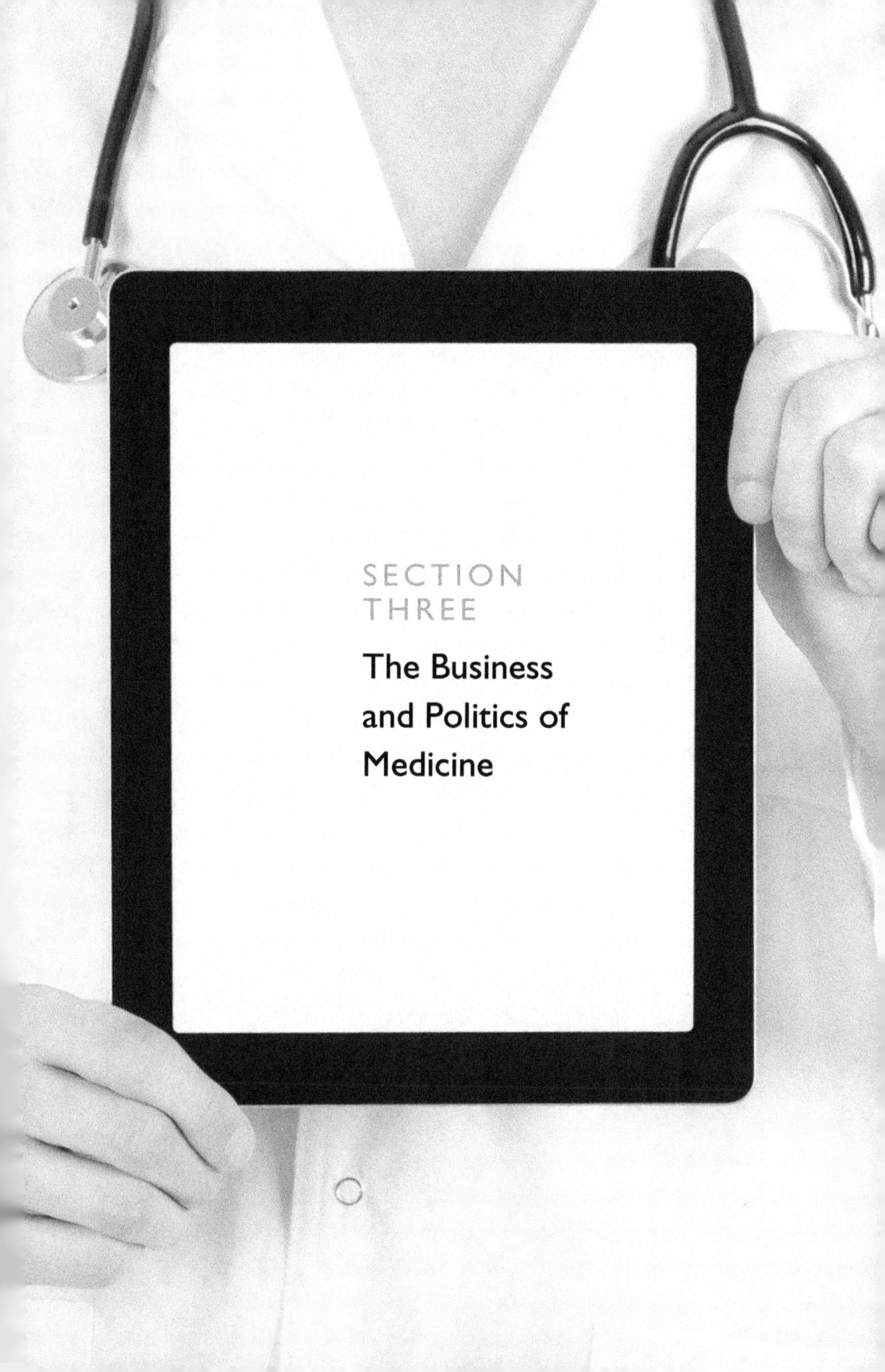

SECTION
THREE

The Business
and Politics of
Medicine

Transitions in Medicine

George Thomas, MD, FACC
Past Chair, Department of Professional Regulations, Florida

The Affordable Care Act, commonly referred to as Obamacare, is now the law of the land. Both supporters and opponents of the law agree on one thing: it will change the health care scene for the foreseeable future. The impact of this legislation on patient care and physician practice is still being vigorously debated, but some trends appear inevitable.

While we are blessed with the best quality medical care in the world, our costs have become prohibitively burdensome. Advances in medicine have helped prolong life expectancy and improved the overall treatment of chronic diseases.

A modern-day physician needs to be both medically well informed regarding the specialty he or she practices and should also be business savvy. In addition, he or she should have a good understanding of the politics behind all the new rules and regulations to ensure proper compliance. He or she needs to run a good office, pay attention to the cash flow, participate in many HMOs that have their own stipulations and guidelines, keep patients and referring physicians happy while keeping the costs under control, and always be vigilant to avoid the ever-present threat of malpractice.

The key issue over the next several years will be how to manage the rapid transition from the system I started with over thirty years ago to a new health care delivery and payment system. One big challenge is to get the exchanges running by January 1, 2014, to make medical insurance available to everyone, as many states have kicked the can down the road. The big issue for physician payment and cost control is going to be making changes in how we pay physicians and incentivizing doctors and hospitals to keep people healthy, and at the same time, increasing coordination of care to make sure that people with chronic illnesses do not fall between the cracks. There will be a lot more experimentation and innovation to identify patients at risk for hospitalization and find methods of early intervention. Episode-based payment, bundle payment, or getting to what is called global payment to give doctors and hospitals a lump sum and hold them accountable for outcomes is something actively discussed.

If you are a caregiver in the US, it is possible that reimbursement will be lower on average, as there will be eighteen million additional patients coming in at Medicare rates. There will be more utilization of preventive and ancillary services, some of which can be high margin, as patients have insurance. It is also likely that federal regulatory oversight of physician practice will increase. The "global payments" designed in Washington, DC, will start with Medicare and may be taken up by private insurers as well. If you are a buyer of healthcare, an employer, or consumer, your commercial premium rates are likely to increase, as happened following Romneycare in Massachusetts, the only state in our nation where universal coverage was implemented.

The old way of reducing health care costs was to just reduce payments to doctors and hospitals; it didn't work. The procedure-oriented payment system, the cost and effectiveness of emergency care, the price of prescription drugs, and out-of-control tort system are a few of the many strains on cost control. We are putting more people in the system and expected to do more with less. The true challenge facing American medicine is to create a modernized system that delivers care in a more intelligent way to improve health quality and at the same time save money.

Although these stories you are about to read were written before Obamacare came into existence, they are just as relevant today and illustrate that the doctors have to be business savvy and must have a good understanding of the business and political trends that influence health care administration.

CHAPTER 39

How I Learned to Be a Better Boss

Employees were taking advantage of the author's inexperience and good nature—until he started setting rules.

Like most doctors of my generation, I learned how to run a private practice through trial and error. At first, it was mostly error. While checking on a job candidate, I called the surgeon whose practice she had recently left.

"I can't remember anything about her," he said.

"How come? She worked in your office for a year and quit just a few months ago," I jokingly prodded. His answer surprised me.

"These girls come and go," he replied. "Some aren't so good, and I let them go. I keep the better ones, but most of them leave for greener pastures. It's a revolving door."

As my practice took shape, I had occasion to remember his words. For instance, there was Melissa, who stole from petty cash. (I'm not using real names.) It took me a couple of years to discover her thievery. So much for my business acumen! I didn't have the guts to prosecute her. Sadly, another assistant later told me she had suspected Melissa; she herself left not long afterward, perhaps feeling guilty because she hadn't alerted me.

It was then that I turned over the job of interviewing and reference-checking to my wife, Susheela, with whom I practice. A pediatrician, she has a better understanding of human nature than I do. Even so, we made some mistakes.

Carey, a nurse, held two jobs. Lack of sleep made her constantly tired, disorganized, and irritable during the day. She even napped between patients. We finally asked her which job she wanted to keep, and she opted for the nighttime one.

Sara also moonlighted, as a cocktail waitress. She didn't last long with us either.

Sherry was a good worker, but she had to do everything her way. As a result, she was argumentative and rude. I finally decided not to put up with her ways.

Amiable Janice spent most of her time in our kitchen, eating and socializing. We finally asked her to leave.

Ramona used our office to sell bonsai. As a gardener, she was terrific; as a billing clerk, she wasn't.

Lorraine was a smart receptionist. But perhaps out of laziness, she would tell people we had no time slots open, even when the appointment book was half-empty. My colleagues tell me this is not uncommon. One day, she outright refused to give an appointment to a patient with an automatic implantable cardioverter-defibrillator who'd had a shock and felt dizzy. That got my attention, and Lorraine was soon out the door.

I thought I'd struck pay dirt with the bright young woman who assured me that her life's goal was to work in a physician's office. Within a few months, she was well versed in patient care and insurance billing. Then she up and left for a job with the local country club, which lured her away with a raise of fifty cents an hour.

Not long after her departure, our practice's lawyer stopped by. When I told him about our revolving door, he joked, "Are you running a halfway house?" We got the message and instituted a policy: Every new employee is on probation for three months. The diligent, honest, pleasant workers get to stay; the lazy or sullen ones get to leave. We continue watching and evaluating performance after the probationary period ends. It took several years, but now we've assembled a core group of five full-time and three part-time employees. I haven't had—or wanted—to fire anyone lately.

Assembling a fine staff is one thing; keeping it is another. In a tight job market, we couldn't afford to lose good workers. We also wanted to promote a harmonious, pleasant office atmosphere that would make patients feel welcome.

To help accomplish that, we began offering what colleagues have often called one of the best medical office compensation packages in town. Our employees participate in our pension and profit-sharing plans, as do the three physicians in the office. (Along the way, we added another cardiologist.) The profit-sharing arrangement is an incentive to be efficient.

Our staff's fringe benefits include life, disability, and health insurance. One staffer didn't need the medical coverage, since she was already covered by her husband's employer. So we gave her a substantial part of the premium we would have paid for her. It pleased her immensely.

Other benefits include pay for unused vacation, sick days, or personal time off, and small cash gifts to employees' children when they graduate or earn an honor. And for several years, we've given a Christmas cash bonus, which is based on seniority. Last year we instituted a productivity bonus, as well, based on the overall increase in practice income.

Just as important as money is the knowledge that we doctors take an active hand in practice management. People want to have rules and oversight; they need to know what's expected of them and how well they're doing. If you don't pay attention to what's going on, employees lose confidence in you. And when you let things slide, they can go downhill very quickly.

So every Wednesday is "employee appreciation day." My wife, who acts as practice manager and office coordinator, orders a pizza lunch with various side dishes. These get-togethers allow the staff to talk about problems that may have surfaced, including differences of opinion about what task is whose job. Airing these differences helps us put down minor skirmishes before they become major clashes. Mostly, though, these sessions are friendly, and everyone looks forward to them even though, with many of the staff on a diet, there's been less pizza lately.

In addition to our Wednesday lunches, we celebrate Secretaries Day and National Nurses Week with lunch at a nice restaurant. At Thanksgiving, everyone gets a turkey, or a coupon for one. Christmas is the occasion for dinner at a posh restaurant or country club. There I thank our employees for their good work, and hand out the bonus checks.

During the workday, we're careful to avoid making disparaging or ego-crushing remarks about the staff. Management experts warn that subtle but painful incivilities take a big toll on morale, and the employer pays for it.

We also show appreciation by soliciting employees' ideas. Every month, at a meeting with the staff and our practice accountant, we review explanations of medical benefits, selected at random, to see whether claims are being coded properly. We also examine the state of accounts receivable.

We rely on employees to tell us whether a temporary worker is needed to increase collections. We prefer to handle cyclical upswings in work volume this way, rather than hiring too many people and then laying off redundant workers during downswings. This policy creates job security for our core group—which they greatly appreciate.

And we listen to employees' ideas for improvements, such as a system to deal with patient complaints. If a patient complains about an interaction with a staffer, my nurse, my wife, or I will call the patient promptly. We also get occasional complaints from patients who don't recall receiving a service, usually because they were recovering from surgery and weren't fully conscious at the time. Billing inquiries go directly to the office manager.

The system works; our patients seem quite happy. While I'd kept reading in business magazines, including *Medical Economics*, that I should be conducting a patient satisfaction survey, I was afraid of what I might find out. Finally, an MBA student approached me and volunteered to do a market analysis of our practice.

He left questionnaires for patients to complete, and also mailed out a few. He tabulated the responses and sent me his recommendations. Although I got high marks in most areas, a couple of patients faulted me for not spending enough time with them. Since getting these results, I try to do more listening. It seems to have paid off; while our census hasn't doubled, it hasn't diminished either.

There's one thing we permit—but don't encourage—our staff to do: take a lunch hour. It's annoying to call a colleague and get a message like this: "Our office is closed and will reopen at two. If this is an emergency, please call 911." Well, calling 911 won't help me when I'm phoning about a patient.

So our office is open continuously from nine to five, and people are expected to stay around and answer phones even when they take a break to eat. Our kitchen has a refrigerator and pantry stocked with healthy food, and employees take turns bringing in food to share. So there's seldom a reason to leave the office.

With plenty of good food and camaraderie here, why would they want to go anywhere?[39]

---

[39] Reprinted with permission from *Medical Economics*: August 7, 2000, 77:13 pg1 12. *Medical Economics* is a copyrighted publication of Advanstar Communications, Inc. All rights reserved.

CHAPTER 40

My Patients Got an HMO to Take Me Back

But did the author win the battle, only to lose the war?

When I returned to my office from a two-week vacation in the summer of 1999, a nasty surprise awaited me. A large Medicare HMO, ProHealth (not its real name), had decided to terminate me and my partner, giving us the required two months' notice. A quick check on our office computer revealed that I was going to lose 440 patients, or about 15 percent of my practice.

I called ProHealth's provider relations supervisor immediately. He gave no explanation for the decision to drop me beyond an oblique reference to "business reasons." When pressed further, he offered that ProHealth was "consolidating" its position in our county and would be contracting with only one hospital and just a handful of specialists.

In talking to my peers, I discovered that a mass de-selection had taken place. ProHealth had terminated three-quarters of its cardiologists as well as many vascular and cardiac surgeons, gastroenterologists, and pulmonary specialists. Local newspaper stories and my HMO contacts suggested that ProHealth was planning to pull out of the county, or at least scale back its involvement here. The word was that it was losing millions of dollars on its local Medicare business.

Why had I been dropped while other cardiologists had been retained? When I contacted the area manager of ProHealth, he told me that I didn't do enough volume in the hospital that was still participating with the plan. I knew that was untrue, since I was quite active in that hospital. I also knew I had treated my patients very well, and that my care was comparatively cost-efficient. Perhaps ProHealth had simply picked a few cardiologists who were willing to give the plan a good financial deal, I told myself.

Nevertheless, I wasn't ready to give up. As the effective date of my termination approached, I mobilized support among colleagues and patients. First, I asked a few of my referring family physicians (FPs) to write letters to ProHealth about the quality of my work. All of them did. I thought this would be effective because the plan wanted to keep its FPs happy.

Next, I composed a form letter for my patients to sign and mail to ProHealth. A number of patients had expressed sympathy for me, and some were really upset that they'd have to choose another cardiologist. So I had my staff call a dozen patients I felt especially close to, and they all obliged.

At the same time, my partner and I urged our ProHealth patients to switch back to traditional Medicare. Alternatively, they could have moved to another Medicare HMO that we belonged to. But there were rumors that that plan, too, might be pulling up stakes, and I didn't want my patients herded around like cattle.

On the other hand, I knew it would be difficult for elderly patients on a fixed income to return to traditional Medicare, because it would mean losing their HMO-subsidized drug benefit and other things Medicare doesn't pay for. One patient with chronic heart failure told me, "I don't want to go to any of the cardiologists still listed on ProHealth's panel. But I can't afford these expensive medications, and I'm on six of them." So he stayed with the plan, although he wrote a strong letter on my behalf.

In the end, I lost all but about thirty of my ProHealth patients. Although that's a small number, I regarded it as a victory, because some of my patients were willing to listen to me.

After my termination in September, I continued to treat ProHealth patients who asked for me when they were in the hospital or the ER. The plan had no problem with paying me for those services. It also paid me to do transesophageal echocardiograms, since I'm one of only three local cardiologists who do the procedure regularly.

But, despite my continued entreaties, ProHealth refused to reinstate me. Not even a recommendation from the CEO of the hospital swayed the plan. Then one day, I heard that a couple of other specialists had been reinstated, and, a bit later, I received a credentialing form from ProHealth. Soon I was participating in the plan again.

It turned out to be a short-lived triumph. Few of my former ProHealth patients returned to me; they had found other physicians and didn't want to leave them. And not long afterward, ProHealth finally left the county. The HMO to which ProHealth had sold its patient "lives" also announced its intention to depart. That would leave the county virtually free of Medicare-managed care. But local residents and their legislative representatives protested. Now, other plans have come in, and I'm getting on their panels. How could I not?

The plain fact is that HMOs are here to stay. No cardiologist in my area can stay in practice with nothing but fee-for-service revenue from traditional Medicare and Blue Cross Blue Shield. So we have to participate in the HMOs and stay in their good graces. Yet I feel I struck a small blow against managed care companies that toss us to the winds whenever it suits them.

The plans don't treat patients very well either when they walk away from some areas because it suits their purposes. But one thing I learned from this experience is that insurers will listen to patients when they stick up for their doctors—especially Medicare patients, who are free to switch plans. They know that if they make a patient unhappy, and the patient starts spreading rumors, he or she will leave the HMO, and others may leave too. So if a plan drops you and you want to be reinstated, your most powerful weapon is your patients.[40]

[40] Reprinted with permission from *Medical Economics*: March 5, 2001, 78:5 pg 118. *Medical Economics* is a copyrighted publication of Advanstar Communications, Inc. All rights reserved.

CHAPTER 41

Unintentional Comments… Undesirable Results

One of the basic dictums in medico-legal jargon is, "never do finger-pointing at the failure of another doctor."

A long-established relationship with a patient and a good rapport with the family can certainly help you to withstand a crisis. On the other hand, a very enthusiastic academic colleague who tells the patient and relatives that a finding was missed in a previous X-ray can pave the way for a malpractice suit. And it did. The story of Robert Stillwell and his wife Melanie (not their real names) is a classic example.

Robert, seventy-three years old, a patient of mine for fifteen years with well-controlled hypertension, presented one day with palpitations from a new onset atrial fibrillation. The diagnosis was sick sinus syndrome with tachy-brady arrhythmias. A permanent pacemaker was implanted and along with medications, and he remained well. He came regularly for his follow-up and occasionally needed treatment for respiratory infections. He had a history of thirty pack years of cigarette smoking but promised to quit.

A couple of years later Robert developed a mini stroke, often called TIA (transient ischemic attack) in medical parlance. As expected, being a smoker, he had severe blockage of the left carotid artery that needed a carotid endarterectomy. He stopped smoking and was doing well but then he had an episode of syncope. Again, he went through complete workup but nothing significant turned up. The pacemaker tested normal and the chest X-ray was unremarkable. But he had developed a right carotid stenosis this time for which he promptly underwent surgery, a right carotid endarterectomy. Once again, he was back to his usual self and enthusiastically resumed his work as a photojournalist.

One day, he presented to the emergency department (ED) with sudden left-sided chest discomfort. I had seen him in the office only two weeks earlier for an acute tracheobronchitis that responded to antibiotics. So I was surprised to see him in the ED. Clinical examination was unremarkable, and he didn't have any evidence of a heart attack, but the chest X-ray report was: "Hyperinflated lungs with some infiltrate in the left hilar area."

The working diagnosis at this stage was COPD and possible bronchopneumonia. With intravenous antibiotics and fluids, he improved. The consulting pulmonologist worried about the possibility of a left hilar tumor. CEA (a marker for malignancy in the body) was significantly elevated at 130. Although the bronchoscopy showed no endobronchial lesion to suggest cancer, a CT scan of the chest showed a seven-centimeter mass in the left hilum, with contiguous left hilar adenopathy, suggestive of a tumor.

A thoracic surgeon, Dr. Thomas, was consulted. The surgeon went back and looked at the chest X-rays done ten months ago and determined that there was, indeed, a subtle abnormality in the left hilum, which most likely represented the beginning of the tumor, although the radiologist had reported "no significant abnormality." He showed both the films to Melanie and discussed these findings, and she became upset. During the next visit to my office, Melanie brought both films for my review. She put them up on my view box and pointed at the shadow in the X-ray, saying: "See this; this is where Dr. T said was the 'beginning of the tumor' a year ago."

Hindsight being 20/20, if you placed both films side by side, one could argue that there may have been a soft, relatively inconspicuous shadow in the first film, which even the radiologist didn't think was significant. I personally looked at the film, and I didn't think I could have made the correct diagnosis at the initial presentation.

Robert underwent a left thoracotomy, which showed a large left hilar tumor with invasion of pericardium, needing extensive surgery—resection of the tumor, attached phrenic nerve, and part of the pericardium with reconstruction, but he succumbed after a stormy postoperative course.

Melanie reviewed all the hospital reports and decided to sue the radiologists who interpreted the X-rays, based on the surgeon's comments. The discovery process continued for two years. They scheduled two depositions for me but the lawyer kept postponing. I dreaded them even though I was not being sued. There is always the fear that after the depositions, the lawyer can change his or her mind and include you in the suit as well. Plus they could put up both X-rays on the view box side by side and ask me if I would have diagnosed this earlier preventing a delay in treatment.

Then one day, as I walked into my office our office manager, came running to announce the news, "You don't have to go for the deposition; they settled." She had contacted the lawyer's office to ask about the new date for deposition. The plaintiffs and the lawyers for the defendants settled the case out of court for an undisclosed amount.

I reflected on the case and the development of the events for a long time and went back to check all the records including X-ray reports. Although one can be a good Monday morning quarterback, I personally couldn't fault the radiologists for not detecting this lesion earlier. I had discussed the X-rays with both radiologists after the wife brought the two films and pointed out the abnormality in the first film. They said, "No, it would have been extremely difficult to diagnose this lesion ahead of time; it is easier when you have a subsequent film to compare."

If the surgeon was discreet in his remarks about the lesion this legal wrangle could have been avoided. Sometimes we become agents of our own destruction with unintentional words. So we need to be very careful about what we say to the patients, especially if you imply that an error was committed by another doctor. I wonder what happened to the old adage, "Speak no evil…," especially if it didn't serve any purpose at this late stage.

It was certainly a relief that I was not sued, although I felt sad for the radiologists. Part of the reason for not including me was probably that I had a good rapport with the wife and had taken care of both of them for many years. And I certainly didn't feel responsible for any errors in the radiological interpretation, if indeed there were any. Normally I look at all chest X-rays and, the one in question—taken ten months before the final diagnosis—looked normal to me also. Only by comparing one with the other simultaneously, could one have been able to see the difference—truly, a retrospective diagnosis. But we all know that even the perception of a missed cancer is an automatic liability issue.[41]

---

[41] First published in AAPI Convention Souvenir 2009.

CHAPTER 42

One Day in November 2002

Although medicine has advanced significantly over the past several decades, practicing medicine in the current environment has become quite difficult thanks to the many extraneous influences.

Being an early riser, theoretically I should have no problem getting to work on time. But I like to spend a couple of hours in the morning on my own personal matters, mostly reading nonmedical stuff like newspapers, magazines, or library books and checking my e-mail or writing a guest editorial for our local newspapers. This is what I call my "sanity hour."

But as if on cue, I would get a call from the hospital at 8:00 a.m. "Doc, your first exercise stress test is ready," and I spring into action. Then it is all rush-rush. Stress hormones start pouring into my blood stream. My *amygdala* would light up in a PET scan.

The answering service follows with more calls almost immediately: "You have two consults, Thornberg in MCCU with atrial fibrillation, and Jarret in 513 with chest pain."

"OK, not too bad," I mutter to myself. But when I reach the hospital, things take a different shape.

"Dr. N..., stat to MCCU!" The patient was just admitted with low blood pressure and sepsis. I quickly evaluate and shout some orders to the nurse. Meanwhile, the stress lab is getting impatient. I am holding up patients and other doctors too.

After an hour, I start making rounds on my own patients. Fortunately, I have only eight patients in my service. Hendricks has just returned from the cardiac cath lab. He has triple vessel disease and needs surgery. We refer all cardiac surgical patients to the nearby Bayonet Point Heart Institute, but Hendricks wants to go to St. Joseph's in Tampa. However, that hospital is not on his insurance plan! Now I have to convince the insurance company to make an exception. That, I know, will be a long ordeal. Oh, my morning has started well!

The next one, McDowell, was sent back from radiology without completing his scheduled biopsy of lung for a "mass lesion." He became so breathless and his blood pressure dropped, after the IV sedation. Nobody had warned me that I was going to face a fuming wife and a barrage of questions.

"How come it couldn't be done today?"

"We are so eager to know the diagnosis. How quickly can you re-schedule it?"

"He was all right till they dropped that medicine into the IV tube. What happened?"

She fired off questions in a single breath. Cautiously (the malpractice monster baring his teeth at me already!) and without looking upset (that wasn't easy, by the way), I tried to explain things. I didn't think it was a good idea to give her a sermon at this time about his sixty pack years of smoking and spending too much time in beer parlors, the root causes of his current problems.

It was becoming painfully obvious that I was doing less medicine and more social and administrative patchwork this morning. I still had to get through a lot of patient care.

Mrs. Jenson, my next patient, a seventy-two-year-old woman, was admitted with sudden mental changes. When I examined her last night, she almost yanked the stethoscope from my neck. She was agitated and rambunctious. This morning, however, she was a totally different person.

"Hi, I remember you. How are you?" she looked like a paragon of grace and charm. Maybe she has recovered from her confusion, I said to myself. Or was I hallucinating?

"I'm OK. How about you? You seem a lot better."

"Oh, yeah? You know I died last night and went to heaven. You guys brought me back. See what you did!"

There was an angry tone in her senseless babbling. I have heard of out-of-body experiences following a cardiac arrest and successful resuscitation, but Mrs. Jenson didn't have any such crisis. It was a funny coincidence that I was reading *The Lovely Bones*, a recent best seller by Alice Sebold, in which the young girl, Susan Salmon, dies and goes to heaven, observes the goings-on down below from her vantage point, and comes back for a short time.

I turned to the nurse and asked, "What did the neurologist say?"

"Oh, he thinks she had a stroke. The psychiatrist thinks she has an acute psychosis."

This is not the first time I've come across two of my experts having diametrically opposite views. Well, let them fight it out.

Suddenly I heard the page from the ER.

"Your patient Bill Withers is here again, with shortness of breath." Bill is what the nurses call a "frequent flier." His home conditions are terrible, and he comes here more for good food and a little rest. I will have to go to the ER and say hello to my buddy.

Soon I start getting calls from the office: "You know your first three patients are already here. When can you get here? You have two new ones today." Whatever happens, I don't like to keep them waiting. Otherwise the complaints might go all the way to Dear Abby!"

"OK, will come pronto. I guess I will finish the rounds after the office."

About 2:00 p.m., my wife, a pediatrician, practice manager, my Girl Friday, and the conflict mediator among the six staffers we have, all in one, reminds me as I run from one examining room to another, "Hey, you haven't had lunch yet."

At 3:00 p.m., there is a fax from the medical records sitting on my desk. It says, "There are fifty-two incomplete charts in your pile. You have two weeks to finish them, before your privileges are suspended." Good grief, I did all my charts only last week! They seem to multiply like rabbits.

I glance at my watch, it is now 5:00 p.m. I hear Phyllis, my secretary, calling from the corridor. "I am running late, Dr. N…Here," My secretary hands over a piece of paper with her neat handwriting, as she is exiting through the back door at 5:00 p.m. "Ron Shaeffer, Room 358, cardiac arrhythmia, Bernie Renfroe—47, angina tele-annex." The evening work has started even before the morning work is over.

My mail has piled up on the desk, and I quickly look at it. The desk is a mess, full of letters and faxes screaming for attention. But I console myself, "A cluttered desk is a sign of a genius." (My wife is a hard sell on that theory though.) I see a reminder for the Critical Care Committee meeting tomorrow at 7:30 a.m., which I am supposed to chair. There is a chart release request from a long-established patient. He is switching to another insurance company that I don't participate in—money versus loyalty.

A lawyer has asked for records. I recognize the patient's name and didn't think there was any negligence. But these days even a perceived bad outcome is cause enough to initiate legal proceedings. Merck Medco wants me to change some of my prescriptions to their preferred drugs, along with a reminder that physicians should be at the front line of the battle to control drug costs. Then there is a graph of my quarterly performance profile from the hospital. And a chart audit report from a PPO (preferred provider organization), a nonphysician advising me of my shortcomings. To top it off, my malpractice carrier has announced an increase in the premium, again. It just doubled through no fault of mine. I haven't had any malpractice cases against me during the past seven years.

Then there are social obligations to fulfill…fundraisers galore! The annual AHA ball this year is asking a thousand bucks! Another reminder from the Patrolman's Benevolence Fund that my donation this year is still pending! An abused women's shelter is starting its first ever "Awareness

Ball," just $1,000 per sponsor, and the county commissioner has sent a special invite. You know what that means…there are invisible strings attached.

The computer man has finished his update for HIPAA compliance for a hefty charge. The main HMO that I participate in insists that I get prior permission for most of the tests I order in the office. Medicare denied reimbursements on the recent patients who had outpatient stress tests. They always have some excuse or other. My accountant says my take-home salary is only thirty-four cents for each dollar. That much overhead?

Welcome to the modern-day health industry. It seems I am working mainly to pay taxes and insurance premiums, and of course, elevate my blood pressure. For a moment my inner longing for the old-fashioned way of practice—when the doctor-patient relationship was a sacred covenant, and I only had to be a doctor, not a businessman or administrator—became profound. I felt sorry for myself for the umpteenth time that I didn't take an MBA.

By the time I wind up my office, dictation and tons of paperwork, it is already 6:30 p.m.

I am back in the hospital, at the Heart Center. My box is full of unread EKGs, Echos, nuclear scans. Then there was just a sweet reminder from the secretary, "You need to finish all your EKGs today—seventy-two-hour time limit, you know."

At 9:00 p.m., my wife pages me impatiently. "Your supper is getting cold, and I am getting hungry. Are you camping out in the hospital today?" She is the gatekeeper of my health. As I open the door of the only car in the parking lot, I gently glance upward and pray silently: "Oh, Heavenly Father, could I just do the medicine part, and perhaps You can take care of the rest of these hassles. Thank you for your urgent consideration."

I get home exhausted with the sad realization that my life doesn't belong to me anymore. *Where are we going with this modern medical practice?* I wonder.

Yet…

Regardless of all these hassles, as an incorrigible Type A workaholic, I love my profession. I work not just because of the financial rewards, but for the "high," the satisfaction of helping somebody and saving someone's life, for the smile and thank you notes I get from grateful patients. My father has always stressed that the fundamental tenet of medicine is to consider the profession as a life's calling.

Well, if only these outside forces could be kept in check![42]

[42] 2004 First published in AKMG (Association of Kerala Medical Graduates) Convention Souvenir.

CHAPTER 43

What is the Name of Your Malpractice Insurer?

That is the first thing the relatives wanted to know after an elderly woman fell in the author's office. Here is how he avoided litigation.

"Come to the office, right away," Becky, my nurse interrupted the ICU rounds. "Sally fell in the examining room, and I think her hip is fractured."

There was near pandemonium in the office by the time I arrived there. Sally was on the floor, quite short of breath and pale. The nurse was administering oxygen. The office manager had summoned the ambulance crew, who arrived to take her to the ICU.

I leaned close to Sally and said softly, "I'll inform your family. Give me their phone numbers."

But she gave me, between short and difficult breaths, her usual answer. "Oh, don't bother to call my children. I don't think they care much. You are my family, Dr. Nathan. I trust your judgment." We did find a number, though, and notified a daughter.

Sally had sustained a fracture of the left hip. In the ICU, she developed severe congestive heart failure and almost went into cardiogenic shock. Her left ventricular ejection fraction, previously around 35 percent, became further depressed. I had to do an emergency right thoracentesis to take out nearly a liter of pleural fluid. Her diabetes needed closer monitoring and stabilization. She was in atrial fibrillation with rapid ventricular response and BP of 90/60. The rate had to be controlled quickly.

The orthopedic surgeon was very reluctant even to touch her, and the anesthesiologist didn't like the idea of her dying in the operating room. The risk was much too high for surgery. Yet without surgery, Sally would never walk.

Just then, the ICU nurse broke into our consultation. "The relatives are outside. They want to see you."

So finally, I get to see Sally's folks. I'd been her physician for four years and had never had any contact with them. In the conference room, I saw a dozen angry faces. The eldest daughter, who had appointed herself as the spokeswoman, asked abruptly, "Doctor, what is the name of your insurance company?"

When Sally had first come to me, she was frail and looked like living death. She was sixty but appeared to be much older. She was a Medicaid patient from another town where no cardiologist would accept her. I was the new kid in town and, coming from a teaching hospital, I was fascinated with the challenge she offered.

And what a challenge! Sally had chronic rheumatic heart disease. She'd already undergone three mitral valve surgeries, and the most recent valve was dysfunctional. There was severe mitral regurgitation, and her left ventricle had the appearance of an end-stage dilated cardiomyopathy. She was a Type II diabetic and had peripheral and carotid vascular disease. Her severe CHF was complicated by pleural effusion and ascites.

During the next several months, she needed several hospitalizations to pull her out of the many crises. I thought that each admission would be her last, but she was indomitable.

My nurse even delivered diuretics and antibiotics to her home, as she had no money and no reliable transportation. We never got enquiries from any of her relatives, including the daughter whom she said lived with her sporadically. I surmised that her family had long since abandoned her. 'My rotten children' is how she referred to them, when she spoke of them at all.

As if Sally didn't have enough problems, she developed cervical cancer with pelvic metastasis, and I had to use my charm and wit on one of our radiation therapists to accept her as his patient. Initially, she couldn't even lie down long enough for radium implantation, and I had to re-admit her to relieve her pulmonary congestion. Only then, could she complete a course of radiation therapy.

During the last four years, amid many critical care admissions, no family member had enquired about her. Becky and I were her sole guardians, so to say. I liked and respected her almost like my mother, and she was grateful for the attention we showered on her.

"Well, doctor, I asked the name of your insurance company."

"Don't you want to know how your mother is doing?"

I was boiling inside, but hoped I didn't show it.

"She fell in your office, didn't she?" The tone was accusatory. No one asked how Sally was doing. They obviously hadn't come to thank me for all the care I'd taken of their mother for four years. All they had on their minds was a lawsuit.

The conversation hit a dead end. I learned later the family had contacted a lawyer. I informed my office-liability and malpractice carriers of impending trouble, but I didn't think that I was at fault in any way. With Sally's frail general status and chronic cardiovascular problems, she could have fallen anywhere and even died.

During the next few days, Sally teetered between life and death. The nurses felt that her waiting family didn't care about her daily condition and probably would be delighted if she just conveniently passed away.

With a degree of vengeance, I went to work. I knew the odds were against us to save this lady. We employed hemodynamic monitoring, multiple thoracentesis, after –load reduction, aggressive decongestive therapy, inotropic support, frequent consultations with respiratory therapists, laboratory monitoring , and all other state-of-the-art critical care therapy.

I constantly prayed and once whispered in Sally's ear: "Don't quit on me now." I think she understood what was going on. We were allies against her "rotten children."

During all this, the relatives asked the nurses only one question. "How long can mother last like this?" Although indignant, the nurses were gracious.

The surgeon and anesthesiologist handled their parts very well. At long last, Sally was discharged—on crutches, but walking.

The nurses hailed this as the biggest success they'd seen in recent times. It was a miracle. We gave high-fives to each other.

The lawyers reviewed my office and hospital charts and could find nothing amiss. The office notes were typewritten and I had included comments about the lack of concern of Sally's relatives.

My own lawyer later reported that the family contacted three trial lawyers who refused to accept the case. One of the daughters even hinted that Sally may have been pushed from the examining table but this didn't stand up to the most rudimentary questioning. Sally, of course, would hear nothing of a malpractice suit against me. She even gave an unofficial statement to the nurses that her falling in my office was entirely her fault.

Finding that they couldn't collect from my insurance company the family dumped Sally back in her small house and went their own way. We had arranged a home-health-care agency to look after her. As an unexpected act of kindness to me, the family transferred Sally's records to another cardiologist.

I miss Sally, but I get a chuckle when I picture her sitting in a chair and flipping the TV channels, fully alive and enjoying whatever life is left for her. She must have a chuckle too, having beaten the odds and given her children a lesson they'll never forget. [43]

[43] Reprinted with permission from *Medical Economics*: September 11, 1996, 72: 17 pg 99–107. *Medical Economics* is a copyrighted publication of Advanstar Communications, Inc. All rights reserved.

CHAPTER 44

My Reputation Went up for Grabs on the Malpractice Bargaining Table

In settling a negligence suit, the author learned that clinical quality counted for nothing. The negotiations were all about money.

In my three decades as cardiologist, I've always taken pride in being a good communicator. And I've always been meticulous—to the point of compulsiveness—about my patients' care. So my first malpractice suit, in 1995, struck me like a fist in the face.

It started the day sixty-seven-year-old Ken Butler came to my office. He'd developed angina four years before, and his pain had worsened. After his exercise stress test came back strongly positive, I recommended a cardiac catheterization. He reluctantly agreed.

During the exam, I noticed a whisper-quiet carotid bruit and ordered ultrasound studies. Performed four days later, the tests showed bilateral occlusion in the 70–80 percent range. Because there were no symptoms, I judged that the bruit didn't warrant urgent attention. I wrote up my notes, my transcriptionist typed them, and they went into the patient's file.

From the cath lab to the OR—rapidly

Butler canceled his first catheterization appointment, but went through with the procedure a few days later. James Thompson who did the catheterization, phoned me from the lab. Butler had severe coronary disease, including the left main coronary, Thompson said. He needed immediate coronary bypass surgery.

I felt confident that after the operation—which was performed in another hospital—Butler's condition would improve.

It didn't. The surgery itself went well, but the next day, the surgeon, David Nichols, phoned me to say that Butler had suffered a stroke. He couldn't speak or walk. And his disabilities were expected to be permanent.

"I didn't know that this patient had had a carotid duplex in your office," he said with tension in his voice. "Did it show any blockage?"

"I assumed Dr. Thompson discussed the case with you," I replied, deeply upset. I didn't even know who from your group would be doing the surgery."

"If I'd known he had carotid disease," Nichols said, "I would have acted faster after the stroke started."

"How could you have reversed it?" I asked.

He sidestepped the question, "Mrs. Butler is pretty upset," he said. "She seems to think that you failed to inform us about the studies and that they showed he had a significant problem."

He was obviously hinting at a lawsuit, but I wasn't worried about that at this point; I just wanted to know my patient's chances for recovery. I couldn't remember a single patient in the last fifteen years who'd suffered a stroke after coronary artery bypass. The surgery had been urgent. I doubted that Butler's asymptomatic carotid disease would have made any difference in the decision to proceed.

Would my insurance coverage be enough?

"Negligence." That's what Butler's lawyer called it in a letter I received several months later.

The lawyer didn't spell out where he thought negligence had occurred, but he asked for a startling amount of information, including copies of "each and every document in your possession" relating to Butler, copies of all my medical contracts and insurance policies, a list of all my business affiliations, and a list of everyone in my office who had ever talked to the Butlers.

I was furious and hurt. For weeks I couldn't sleep. I felt as if black clouds had settled directly over my head and would stay there for months, perhaps years. My malpractice was hardly reassuring. "A verdict in excess of your policy limits is highly possible," read the letter from John May, the insurance executive who was handling my case. "Therefore, you may wish to have your personal attorney associate with us in your defense."

A personal attorney? I'd kept my coverage below $1 million, as did many of my colleagues, so I wouldn't be a target for lawsuits. Apparently my strategy had backfired. I contacted a private attorney, Dick Beasley, who informed me that he charged $200 per hour and would require a one-time retainer of $2,000!

Sidney Hackett, the insurance company attorney who would be taking my case, suggested I wait to see how the suit developed before I hired my own lawyer. I took the advice.

Preparing for a game of blame-slinging

My second letter from the plaintiffs' lawyer came several weeks later. In it were thirty intimidating questions and demands.

"Please describe in detail any and all discussions you had with Dr. Nichols relating to Mr. Butler, regardless of whether the discussion was before or after Mr. Butler's surgery," was one. The lawyer also wanted to know, "Do you contend any person or entity other than you is, or may be, liable in whole or in part for the claims asserted against you in this lawsuit?" And I was instructed to provide my "entire educational background" and "entire professional background."

In responding, I was careful not to point a finger at anyone. Hackett edited my comments so they were strictly on point, explaining, "We don't want to give them any ammunition.

Soon I received the first of a flurry of letters from Hackett and May. Or, rather, I got copies of letters they were sending to each other about the case. They called each other "Sonny" and "Johnny."

It got so I was almost afraid to open my mail. I learned from one seven-page letter that the allegations of my "negligence" stretched for about a mile. My heart sank as I read that the claims included "failure to examine, evaluate, diagnose, and treat" Butler's condition. Under oath, Mrs. Butler had testified that I hadn't even examined her husband during his first visit to my office, when I'd first heard the bruit. I was shocked to the core.

In a letter from Sonny to Johnny, I learned, surgeon Nichols had said he should have been informed of Butler's carotid disease so he could have told the Butlers it increased the risk of stroke with the surgery.

I wondered: Wouldn't Nichols have seen the patient's chart before the operation? Or wouldn't Thompson, who performed the catheterization, have read the chart and told Nichols about the carotid disease? The Butlers didn't know the results of the studies; they'd never called my office. And I hadn't called them because an asymptomatic bruit, even one with a 70-80 percent occlusion, was news that I felt could wait for the next appointment.

Hackett said he expected a lot of blame-slinging about the lack of communication on the carotid – disease studies. It was clear to me by now that a single phone call to any of these parties would have saved my neck.

In the meantime, the plaintiffs wanted 2.5 million from the doctors and the hospital combined. And the plaintiffs' attorney wanted to know if I had any insurance I hadn't told him about.

"Friendly" testimony is hardly reassuring

The depositions that preceded me were harrowing. Even my own expert witness, a cardiologist, was a mixed blessing.

"No physician other than Dr. Nathan appreciated the bruit," he testified. Then he added rhetorically, "I concur that Dr. Nathan may be at fault" in the communication of information about the patient. As Hackett put it in a letter, "He is implicitly critical of the case." So much for support!

A neurologist also testified, saying that patients with critical stenosis should have a carotid endarterectomy first, followed by a bypass, or else have combined surgery. I felt he didn't understand the specific situation: I'd had to OK emergency surgery.

Thompson, in his deposition, said that he had expected me to tell him about the carotid disease verbally, even though my office had sent him copies of the charts.

The tide began to turn, it seemed to me, when Nichols gave his deposition. Despite the cost to him, the surgeon candidly testified that he hadn't tried to get more information from Thompson, the referring cardiologist. He said he hadn't heard a bruit himself. His comments suggested that he wouldn't have done a combined surgery in any case, because it would have entailed a high risk of stroke.

Further, Nichols refused to say whose responsibility he thought it was to relay the information. In Hackett's words, "With the plaintiffs' counsel practically begging him to criticize Nathan and Thompson for failing to tell him about the carotid disease, Nichols adamantly refused to blame the other physicians."

A video destined to move a jury

When Mrs. Butler finally gave her deposition, it was horrifying. Her husband couldn't speak, walk, or swallow. He was incontinent. He suffered mood swings. And he was entirely dependent on Mrs. Butler. She couldn't leave the house unless an aide was able to sit in for her.

To illustrate the point, the lawyers had made a two-hour videotape titled "One Day in the Life of the Butlers." I didn't see it, but the lawyers suggested it would have squeezed tears from a brick, let alone a jury.

Faced with the video, my insurer wanted to mediate rather than go to trial. But I was still grappling with the case on a personal level. Why wasn't anyone recognizing my prompt diagnosis and careful management?

Hackett's comments summed it up. "If it weren't for your clinical skills, you wouldn't even have been involved in this case," he said one day. "If you hadn't recorded the bruit that everyone else missed there might not have been a malpractice case at all." The irony was almost too much to bear.

May again reminded me that a settlement might exceed my policy limit. Reluctantly, I phoned attorney Dick Beasley and told him I needed his help.

Bargaining in the malpractice marketplace

Mediation day arrived.

"How long will this take?" I asked John May as the elevator rose to the twenty-eighth floor of a skyscraper.

"How long is infinity?" he deadpanned, before adding, "Anywhere from two to twenty hours."

In a boardroom with a glorious view of Tampa Bay, the twelve of us, defendants and layers, took our places around a long conference table. Mrs. Butler gazed, expressionless, out the window.

The mediator, Larry Berger, started out by stating that the facts were to be communicated through counsel—in other words, the rest of us were to keep silent. It wasn't easy after the lead plaintiffs' attorney got going. He went on and on about the miseries the Butlers were suffering, bearing heavily on the theme that a communication breakdown among physicians was the source of their pain. In fact, the plaintiffs' attorneys focused their case not on medical judgment itself, but on the lack of communication and its detrimental effect on medical judgment.

The attorneys for the defendants emphasized that knowing about the asymptomatic carotid bruit wouldn't have affected the way Butler was treated.

After that, the defendants and their lawyers went to one room, Mrs. Butler and her lawyers to the other. Berger, the mediator, joined us.

"How do you think a jury will react when they see an invalid stroke patient in a wheelchair?" he asked.

"The surgery was urgent. We had no choice," said Hackett.

"Do we agree that the problem was communication?" Berger asked.

Beasley butted in. "You read the depositions; there was a real problem in communication. No one will come away unscathed." My personal counsel was weakening my position, and he was charging my $200 an hour to do it.

May, who held the insurer's purse strings, volunteered that, although the case was perfectly defensible, he would offer $100,000 to settle it.

Mediator Berger went to the next room and was back almost before the door had closed. "Counteroffer is $2.4 million," he announced.

"No way," said May.

The defense lawyers dickered. "We will open a trial with a statement about communication. It'll be a big hit with the jury," said one. "Offer $850,000 and settle for $1.5million," said another.

"With a $2.5 million potential verdict, offering $100,000 is an insult." interjected Beasley. My own attorney didn't seem eager to defend me at trial.

May, a shrewd businessman, knew how to haggle. As the day went on, he kept offering slightly more and the plaintiffs kept demanding slightly less, while Berger shuttled between the two rooms.

It was no different from the bargaining I'd seen at a country market. I began to realize that this case—not to mention my reputation and peace of mind and that of the other doctors—was to these lawyers exactly what a basketful of tomatoes was to the farmer. Butler's treatment was only the backdrop; mediation was all about money.

Finally, all five defense lawyers unanimously recommended that May settle high, with suggestions ranging from $850,000 to $1.5 million. Put a nice chunk up there, they urged.

But May refused. The session was adjourned around 3:00 p.m.

Trying to avoid finger-pointing

Another flurry of letters followed. Beasley's was dated the very next day.

"Yesterday's mediation was a disappointment, given May's unwillingness to offer the kind of money to effectuate an amicable settlement," he wrote. "I remain concerned that a jury would find you to some degree at fault. I would appreciate your accepting my recommendation that you settle."

The next letter was from Hackett to May. Hackett warned that a judgment against me would probably exceed my policy limits. He wanted assurance that I'd be assigned only a small percentage of the blame so my share of the payment wouldn't overshoot my coverage. He wanted the same consideration for a settlement.

A letter from the plaintiffs' attorney pointed out that, in addition to the Butlers' plight, having the doctors point fingers at one another at trial would give the case plenty of "sizzle." He wanted to settle, and hinted that he might make a "policy-limits demand" against me. In other words, he'd settle for every penny of insurance I had.

The letter left me oddly relieved. My ordeal might at last be coming to an end.

On our second mediation day May started out with an offer of $250,000. The plaintiffs' lawyers countered with $2.4 million—the exact amount of their first counteroffer in the previous day of mediation. We seemed headed for an impasse.

This time, though, May told Berger that he would pay expenses only if they were associated with the incident itself—hospital expenses, for instance, but not home or nursing care. That became a bargaining chip. The other side agreed, and they came down to $2.2 million.

May's stonewalling response was, "Get real." The plaintiffs came down to $1.95 million.

May next asked for the hospital's lawyer, who had joined in the mediation but was sitting alone in a separate room.

"Well?" May asked as the lawyer entered.

"Our error is only 5 percent," said the hospital lawyer. "That's all we have."

"Bye-bye," said May sarcastically.

Berger took the details to the plaintiffs and returned, "OK, they're down to $1.5 million now—for you guys only. Not the hospital."

May shot back. "How about $325,000?"

Berger disappeared again.

The strain of the parley was getting to me. May turned and said to me, "These are mom-and-pop cases. You know that, don't you? Naturally, the family is angry—they never think they share any blame."

Berger returned. "They're negotiating with the hospital," he said. "They came down to $1.47 million from the three doctors."

"That's not realistic," May responded. "Hey, I offered a quarter of a million just to open it up this morning."

A few minutes later, they had come down to $1.3 million.

Over the next three hours, Berger got a lot of exercise. There were offers and counteroffers and counteroffers. At one point, the plaintiffs said they'd release me from the suit if they got $1.25 million from other doctors. The surge of relief that I felt lasted only as long as it took May to turn it down. When May raised his offer to $450,000, the plaintiffs offered to accept $1 million from the surgeon and to release the other doctors. May again said no.

May was wearing the plaintiffs down. At the same time, he was working on the hospital's lawyer, convincing him that the hospital had more exposure than he'd thought.

Finally, just after 5:00 p.m., Berger came back from the plaintiffs' room with a smile on his face.

"We are done!" he said. A settlement had been reached for an amount both sides agreed to keep confidential.

Hackett later told me that the lawyers had together described that my "error" was 1.5 percent of the case. At that moment, I felt as if the black clouds that still hung over my head had begun to lift.

I learned a lot from this difficult episode. A dire emergency and a small gap in communication had brought this malpractice case into being. Just one more phone call, one or two more sentences spoken to the other doctors, and the case would have never happened.

Eventually, I decided to increase my malpractice coverage. I don't ever want to have to compromise my professional reputation again by settling when I'm innocent of the charges.

And I don't ever again want to see my reputation haggled over as if it were a basket of produce in a country market.[44]

[44] Reprinted with permission from *Medical Economics*: August 10, 1998, 75: 15 pg 51–66. *Medical Economics* is a copyrighted publication of Advanstar Communications, Inc. All rights reserved.

CHAPTER 45

Prompt Attention

All types of patients come to the hospital emergency room for treatment. Keeping them happy will go a long way in preventing litigation.

Only after becoming the chair of the Quality Assurance Committee in one of our hospitals, did I realize how difficult and at times daunting a task it is. You have to criticize the performance of your colleagues, send tough letters (although I try to couch them with a lot of polish), and then read their defensive, at times a bit nasty, responses. Often I end up apologizing to them instead of dictating terms from my vantage point. Much worse are the letters from patients who are critical about the treatment they received in the hospital ER or other areas or the performance of *this* doctor or *that* nurse or something similar. Of course, if there are any differences of opinion between doctors or doctors and nurses, they also get sent to this committee.

The following real-life story unfolded with a letter of complaint written to the CEO of our hospital and channeled to me for action. I tried to dig into the case and in that process interviewed many people to get precise information and the basis of the complaint. Here is the reconstructed story, incorporating all the details.

Steven Parker was looking forward to his day off. He had wanted to do some badly needed repairs on his vintage car. He always liked tinkering with the costly toy in the garage. This day was set aside for an expression of his creative talents.

He had just opened the hood of the car and started looking at the engine. Suddenly a frantic call came from the backyard. "Honey, Jessica fell from the swing and is bleeding from her lip. You better take her to the ER right away," Molly, his wife, cried out.

"Oh, no, not today!" Steven was talking more to himself. He wanted to finish the repair job.

"Won't take a minute. The cut looks small," Molly said consolingly, as she brought the four-year-old Jessica indoors.

The hospital parking lot was nearly full. After driving around for a full five minutes, Steven found a spot in the far corner. As he came close, he was disappointed to find the "disabled" sign. There were more signs, like "reserved for the clergy," "for maternity patients only," and so on. Luckily, a woman pulled out, and he rushed to grab the spot, nearly hitting her car. She gave him a look.

The ER waiting room was overflowing with patients. There was a queue in front of the registration counter. Jessica hadn't stopped crying after the fall. The cut was still bleeding. Steven peeked through the glass panels at the entryway. It was a busy little place. All the stretchers in the corridors were occupied. "Today must be my lucky day." Steven sighed. "I don't know when I will get out of this place." He wrote "Jessica Parker" in the sign-in sheet and impatiently waited for his turn.

"Could somebody attend to this little girl right away, please?" Steven asked politely, after waiting for a few minutes.

"Not to worry, have a seat." One of the volunteers reassured him. "It won't be too long."

With difficulty, Steven found a seat and put Jessica on his lap. She was still moaning and groaning. He didn't see any triage nurse around. The registration clerk, relaxing like a royal scion, was quite oblivious of the situation.

"Hey, listen," Steven demanded as he walked up to the counter tapping his watch. He had been waiting for a full fifteen minutes. "What is the delay? I don't have all day, you know." He couldn't take this silent neglect anymore.

"What is your name, sir?" the clerk politely asked in her typical southern drawl.

"I am Steven Parker. My daughter Jessica has cut her lip and it is still bleeding."

"OK, Mr. Parker, please fill out these forms. Somebody will attend to her soon."

"I wish you had given me these forms earlier." Steven was getting a little edgy now. His mind was still on the unfinished job in the garage.

"OK, you can go in now," the clerk beckoned to Steven after a few minutes. "The nurse will ask a few questions and the doctor will see you soon."

Once inside, Steven looked around. There was plenty happening there. Life's wonderworks were on full display. A car accident victim was getting a blood transfusion. The constant "heaving sound" of an artificial respirator was a powerful reminder that somebody's life was hanging in a precarious balance. Two nurses were hurriedly attending to a man who looked ashen and was clutching his chest. There were a few parents and children too, trying to console each other. The place looked more like a battlefield with many wounded.

Steven had to answer a battery of questions from the nurse, and after what seemed to be an eternity, the doctor finally materialized. Steven wasn't in a mood to answer the same questions again but decided to co-operate for fear of losing more time. He wanted to avoid a last-minute showdown. He was still hoping to get back to his house soon and continue working on his car. The doctor examined Jessica. Suddenly, there was a look of concern on his face.

"Did you notice Jessica's tooth is very loose? It is nearly dislodged from the socket."

"Oh, my! What do we do now?" Steven wasn't quite ready to face this new problem.

"We have to consult the oral surgeon, Dr. Pilkington, who is on call today."

"How long is that going to take?"

"Maybe a few minutes. In the meanwhile I will stitch up this wound," the doctor reassured him. Attending to the lip turned out to be a simple matter. But there was no sign of the oral surgeon.

"Did you hear from Dr. Pilkington?" Steven asked the nurse after a while.

"Oh, didn't the doctor tell you? Dr. Pilkington is out of town. Dr. Kory is covering for him. He hasn't called back yet."

Steven's face became livid.

"I have already spent nearly three hours in this goddamn ER. What kind of a joint are you running here?" He was ready to explode.

"Hey, watch your words, mister. Don't you see, this place is very crowded today? We are doing the best we can." The nurse appeared somewhat irked, more out of helplessness. She didn't want to prolong the debate.

All this time, little Jessica sat there like a frightened fawn. She was too scared to cry. This was an adult's world, and she dared not enter it. Just then, one of the other nurses came on the scene.

"Mr. Parker, Dr. Kory cannot come to the ER now. But if you take Jessica to his office, he will be glad to fix the tooth."

"And where is his office, may I ask?" Steven's voice was loud and sarcastic.

"Oh, it is about ten miles down the road. We will give you the instructions."

"Why didn't you send me to the dentist in the first place?" Steven's face was aflame with anger.

"If you had told us in the first place that her tooth was loose, you could have gotten to Dr. Kory sooner." The nurse tried to defend herself.

Steven clenched his fists and ground his teeth. He could feel his muscles getting taut. What is this, some kind of game? He wanted to shout a few obscenities, but immediately changed his mind when he saw a cop walking into the ER.

Sensing that it was not good for the hospital to have an irate and vociferous patient, the doctor called Steven aside and decided to make amends. He called Dr. Kory personally and made an emergency appointment to take care of Jessica free of charge and gave the directions to get there. Steven realized that he may have been a little short-tempered and decided to cool down and follow the doctor's directions.

After patiently listening to Steven's complaints and extensive discussion subsequently, we were able to avoid litigation against the hospital. All's well that ends well.[45]

---

[45] First published in AKMG Annual Alaska Cruise Convention Souvenir aboard the *Norwegian Star*, July 2011.

AAPI – American Association of Physicians of Indian origin
AKMG—Association of Kerala Medical Graduates
AHA—American Heart Association
Amiodarone—a drug for treating serious heart rhythm disorders
Amebiasis—infection with the parasite ameba
Analgesic—a pain killer
Anesthesiologist—a physician specializing in giving anesthesia
Aneurysm—widening or ballooning of an artery
Antihelmintic—drugs that treat parasites (worms) from the body
Aortic valve—the valve through which blood from the left side of the heart flows into the aorta
Atrial fibrillation—irregularity of the heart rhythm that originates from the atrial chambers
AV fistula—arterio venous graft for dialysis

BP—blood pressure
BUN—blood urea nitrogen, a determinant of kidney function

CBC—complete blood count
CCU/MCCU—coronary care unit
CEA—carcinoembryonic antigen, a type of protein in the blood of patients with certain types of cancer, a marker for malignancy in the body
COPD—chronic obstructive pulmonary disease
CT scan—computed axial tomography, a special imaging tool to detect internal lesions
CVP—central venous pressure
Cardiac catheterization—a special procedure in which a catheter is threaded into your heart via femoral or brachial artery for evaluation
Cardiomyopathy—a type of heart disease with enlargement of the heart and decreased cardiac muscle function leading to heart failure

Carotid duplex—ultrasound of both carotid arteries in the neck

Carotid endarterectomy—cleaning of the plaque in the carotid arteries

Cath lab—cardiac catheterization laboratory

Chetta—older brother in Malayalam language

Cholecystitis—inflammation of gallbladder

Chondrocalcinosis—pseudogout, caused by deposition of calcium pyrophosphate crystals in the joints

Code (Coding) —medical lingo for cardiac arrest

COPD—chronic obstructive pulmonary disease

Coronary artery—artery that delivers blood to the heart muscle

Creatinine—a determinant of kidney function

D50—dextrose 50 percent solution for intravenous use

DNR—do not resuscitate

ED—emergency department

EKG—electrocardiogram

ER—emergency room

Echocardiogram—ultrasound of the heart

Ejection fraction—the fraction of blood pumped with each beat, a determinant of the pumping ability of the heart.

Electrophysiology—the science of elucidating, diagnosing, and treating cardiac arrhythmias (the electrical activities of the heart)

Emphysema—a chronic lung disease resulting in damage to the alveoli leading to shortness of breath, often from smoking

Endobronchial lesion—a lesion inside the bronchial tube, commonly from tumor

Femoral vein—the large vein in the thigh, used for cardiac procedures

Gout—acute painful inflammatory arthritis caused by elevated levels of uric acid.

Groshong catheter—a central venous catheter often used for dialysis, administration of medicines, etc.

HMO—health maintenance organization

Hemoptysis—coughing up of blood, often mixed with phlegm

Hepatitis—inflammation of the liver, usually produced by a virus

Heparin—intravenous anticoagulant

Heparin Lock—a small tube attached to the vein for IV access

Hepatomegaly—enlarged liver

Hilum—a wedge-shaped depression on the inner surface (or root) of each lung

Hilar prominence—prominent shadow at the root of the lung on the chest X-ray, often raising the possibility of a tumor

Holter monitor—an ambulatory monitor used for recording 24hr EKG

Hyperalimentation—intravenous feeding through a central venous catheter

ICD—implantable cardioverter defibrillator, very useful for patients who suffer from lethal arrhythmias like ventricular fibrillation

ICU—intensive care unit

IMI—inferior myocardial infarction

INR—international normalized ratio, a test that measures the thinning of blood, used for monitoring anticoagulant (like warfarin) therapy

Inotropic—a drug that improves the contractile ability of the heart

Integrelin (Eptifibatide)—an anti-platelet agent that prevents blood clots or heart attack in people with severe chest pain and in patients undergoing angioplasty.

Ischemia—decreased blood flow in the heart muscle, leading to chest pains

LA—left atrium—top chamber on the left upper side of heart

LV—left ventricle—the chamber on the left lower side of heart

Lymphadenopathy—enlarged lymph glands, a sign of inflammation

ma meillure amie—my best friend

MI—myocardial infarction—heart attack

Metastasis—spread of cancer to distant organs

Mitral valve—the valve between left atrium and left ventricle

Mitral stenosis—narrowing of the mitral valve

MRCP magnetic resonance cholangiographic pancreatogram, a scan used for visualization of liver, bile ducts and pancreatic ducts.

O2—oxygen
OR—operating room

PTCA—percutaneous transluminal coronary angioplasty
PET scan—positive emission tomography A PET scan uses radiation, or nuclear medicine imaging to produce 3- dimensional, color images of the functional processes specific organs in the human body.
Parasitosis —infestation with parasites
Pericardium—the outer covering of the heart
Pneumocystis—a type of fungus that produces pneumonia, common in immunosuppressed patients like AIDS patients

Septic arthritis—inflammation of the joints from an infection
Sinus tachycardia—an increase in the heart rate of 100/mt or more, originating from sinus node
Splenomegaly—enlarged spleen, an organ inside the abdomen below the left diaphragm
Stenosis—narrowing of an artery
Syncope—fainting, passing out
Synovial fluid—fluid from inside the joint

TB—tuberculosis
TEE—Transesophageal echo—ultrasound study of the heart through a special tube inserted into the stomach
Tachy—Brady syndrome—a condition associated with slow and fast heart rate
Thallium stress test—stress test for the heart accompanied by nuclear imaging
Thoracentesis—aspiration of fluid from the chest (pleural cavity)
Thoracotomy—opening the chest for surgery

Trendelenburg—a position in which a patient lies face up with his or her feet above the head, often useful for certain procedures

Thrombolytic therapy—clot-dissolving treatment for heart attack

Ventricular tachycardia—a fast heart rhythm that originates in one of the ventricles of the heart and is potentially life-threatening

WBC count—white blood cell count

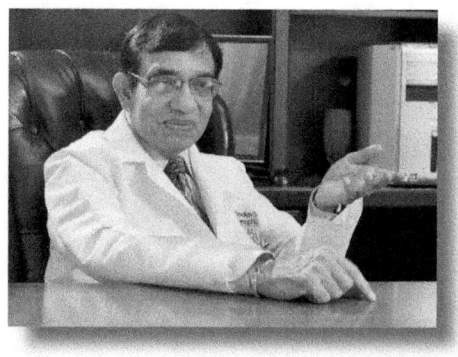

Dr. M. P. Ravindra Nathan, MD, FACC, FACP, FRCP (London & Canada), FAHA

Dr. M. P. Ravindra Nathan is a physician with fifty years of experience in the practice of medicine and cardiology. He was the director of Hernando Heart Clinic in Brooksville, Florida, for thirty years, 1981–2011. Currently he practices cardiology in Hernando County, Florida. He is also an author, speaker, and humanitarian.

Dr. Nathan was born in India and graduated from Trivandrum Medical College, India, and then received his post-graduate medical training in England. He has worked in London, Cambridge, Sheffield, and Sunderland, UK. He came to the United States in 1972.

He is board certified in internal medicine and cardiovascular diseases. He is a fellow of the Royal College of Physicians of London, American College of Medicine, American College of Cardiology, American Heart Association, and Royal College of Physicians of Canada.

He has published more than 180 articles and stories including research papers in scientific journals and lay press. He has been a frequent contributor to *Medical Economics, Cortlandt Forum, Journal of the Florida Medical Association, Tampa Bay Times,* and *Hernando Today,* and he writes a monthly column on medical matters for *Khaas Baat,* an Indian magazine. He was the editor in chief of the *AAPI Journal,* and he is currently its emeritus editor/advisor. He is also the past president of AKMG (Association of Kerala Medical Graduates) and past president of the Hernando division of the American Heart Association.

Dr. Nathan recently edited, along with five other authors, a coffee table volume of 215 pages titled *Archives of AKMG,* which was released on July 13, 2012 in Detroit by AMA president Dr. Jeremy Lazarus.

An interesting collection of essays and real life stories that reflect the many issues, concerns and challenges facing physicians and patients alike in modern day medical practice. Each story is gracefully presented and ends with a moral. Written by an eminent cardiologist, the book is immensely readable and enjoyable by medical and non-medical people alike.

Jayesh Shah MD, Past President, AAPI, San Antonio, TX

This book is a delight to read with such vivid description of personal experiences allowing one to look into the heart of the provider and the patient as they journey through their illness. As a Professor of Nursing this book is a must for students who need to identify with these experiences in order to understand the patient's role. A must read!!!!

Savitri Singh Carlson PhD,

Professor of Nursing, California State University, Long Beach, CA

Reading the book "Stories from My Heart" was an unforgettable experience. Each piece is written with power and passion, and manages to capture the heart of the reader. I believe everybody should read this book.

Chennat Gopalakrishnan MA, Ph.D

Professor Emeritus & Chief Editor, Journal of Natural Resources Policy Research

www.ingramcontent.com/pod-product-compliance
Lightning Source LLC
Chambersburg PA
CBHW051445170526
45166CB00001B/116